"SAY and ___ Holiday Unit Worksheets

Written by Anita K. Robbins and Sara M. Jackson
Edited and Illustrated by Sharon G. Webber

Halloween • Christmas • Easter
George Washington's Birthday
Valentine's Day • Thanksgiving
Abraham Lincoln's Birthday
Hanukkah • St. Patrick's Day
Martin Luther King's Birthday

Lots of reproducible activities, poems, and stories for each holiday!!

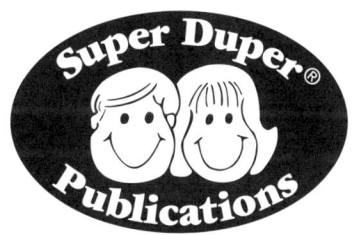

ISBN 1-58650-017-1

www.superduperinc.com
Post Office Box 24997 • Greenville, South Carolina 29616
Call Toll Free 1-800-277-8737 • Fax Toll Free 1-800-978-7379

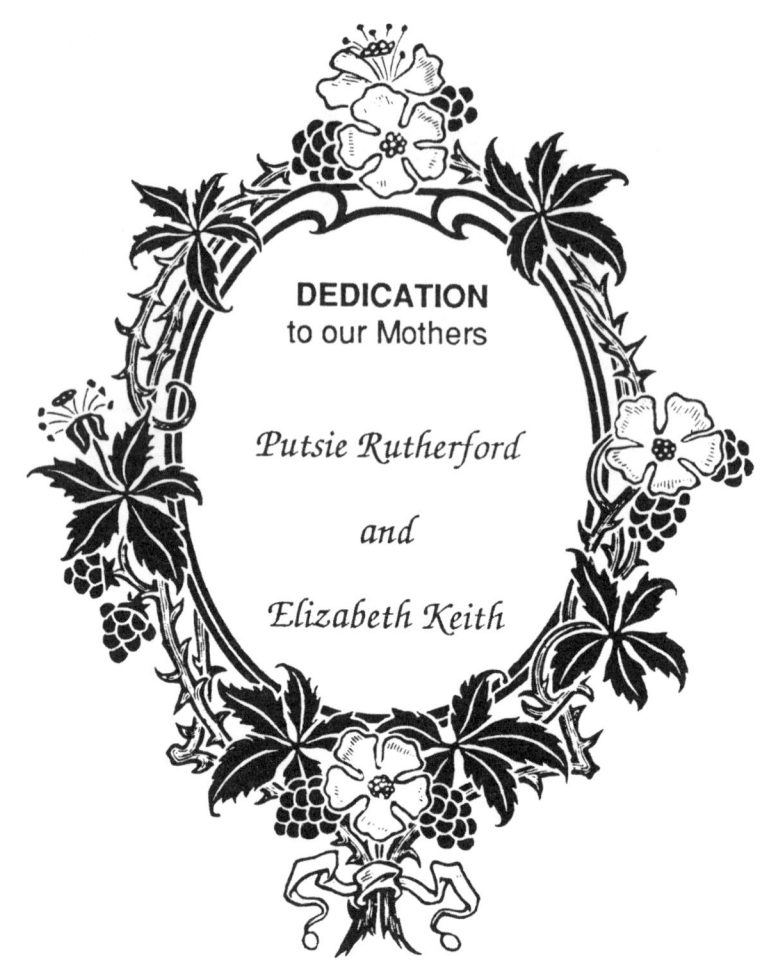

DEDICATION
to our Mothers

Putsie Rutherford

and

Elizabeth Keith

Acknowledgments

The authors would like to thank the following people: LeDhu Stutts
for sharing her Christmas bulletin board ideas. Cathy Massey for
sharing her decoration tree used for various holidays. Laura Sebotnick
for her input on the Hanukkah story. Pam Dixon for typing our first draft.

About the Authors

Sara M. Jackson has a B.S. degree in Speech Pathology from Texas Woman's University. She also holds a M.Ed in Special Education from Converse College. Sara is employed as a speech - language pathologist in Greenville, South Carolina. She is a member of the South Carolina Speech and Hearing Association.

Anita K. Robbins has a B.S. degree in Speech Pathology from East Tennessee State University. She also holds a M.Ed in Special Education from Converse College. Anita is employed as a speech - language pathologist in Greenville, South Carolina. She is also a member of the South Carolina Speech and Hearing Association.

The authors have worked together for 18 years and have shared an interest in children's language development.

About the Illustrator

Sharon G. Webber has a B.S. degree in Speech Pathology from the University of Georgia and she also holds a Master of Speech Pathology degree from the University of South Carolina. She is a member of the American Speech and Hearing Association and the South Carolina Speech and Hearing Association. Sharon is the President of the Super Duper Speech Company in Greenville, South Carolina.

Introduction

These holiday units have been designed to teach young children language concepts by introducing core vocabulary and presenting it in various ways. The holidays are divided into seven sections: Halloween, Thanksgiving, Christmas/Hanukkah, Famous Americans (Washington, Lincoln, King), Valentine's Day, St. Patrick's Day, and Easter.

We want to represent a variety of our language development population. We have attempted to do this in a nonstereotyped manner. The variety of activities have been designed to make learning fun and to save time for you. You may reproduce activities and worksheets as often as needed for classroom use!

Table of Contents

ST. PATRICK'S DAY

EASTER

Let's Talk About Halloween
Halloween - Worksheet 1

Introduction to Halloween

Instructor: Tell the child about Halloween .

Ex: Halloween is a holiday that we celebrate on October 31st. Children dress in costumes. Sometimes costumes look like cats, witches, or ghosts. Children go around their neighborhood "trick or treating." They usually get a lot of candy in their bags.

Core Vocabulary

Use the picture cards (pages 2 and 3) to introduce the Halloween core vocabulary. Have the child color the pictures. The pictures may be cut out and mounted on light cardboard. Describe each picture. Tell about the size, color, particular attributes of each object.

Match-up Activity

Reproduce two of each picture to make a set. Have the child find the matching pictures after you scramble them.

Memory Game

Place two to four cards on the table. Have the child look at the cards for a few seconds. Cover or turn them over. Have the child name the pictures from memory.

Other Suggestions/Activities

- Reproduce the picture cards. Use with gameboard (page 27). Have the child name or describe picture before moving.

- Reproduce two of each picture. Use to play concentration game.

- Place the following cards face down on the table: bat, skeleton, monster, ghost, witch, owl, cat, spider. Have the child choose a picture and then pretend that he is that character.

- Place cards face down on the table. The instructor chooses a picture and begins telling a story about it. Then the child chooses a picture and incorporates the picture into the existing story. Continue taking turns choosing pictures and adding to the story.

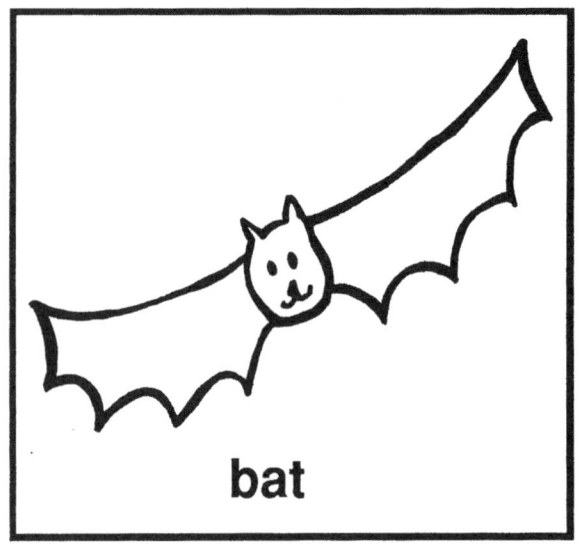

bat

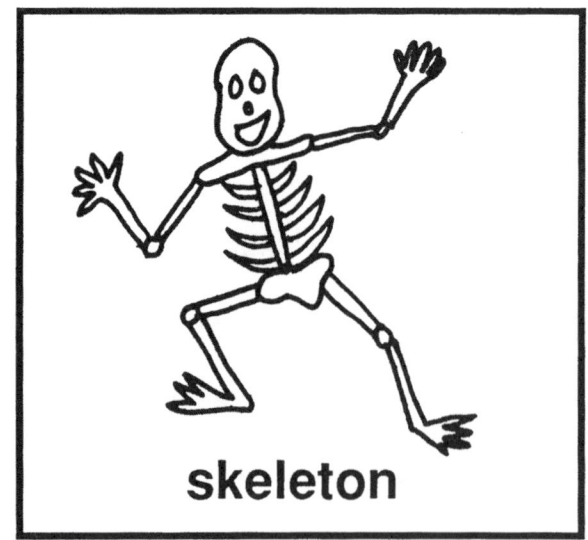

skeleton

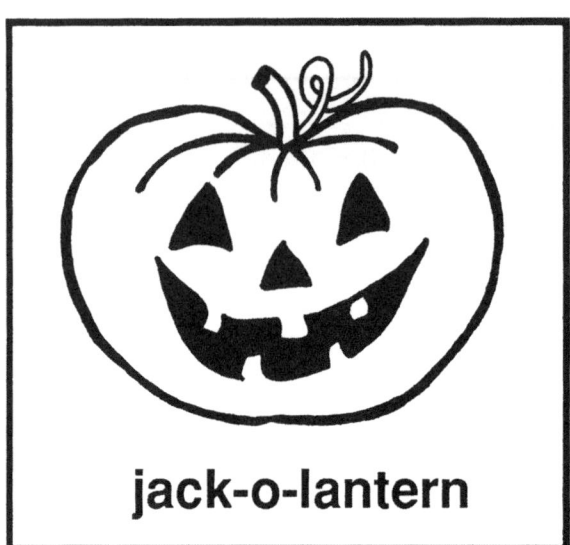

jack-o-lantern

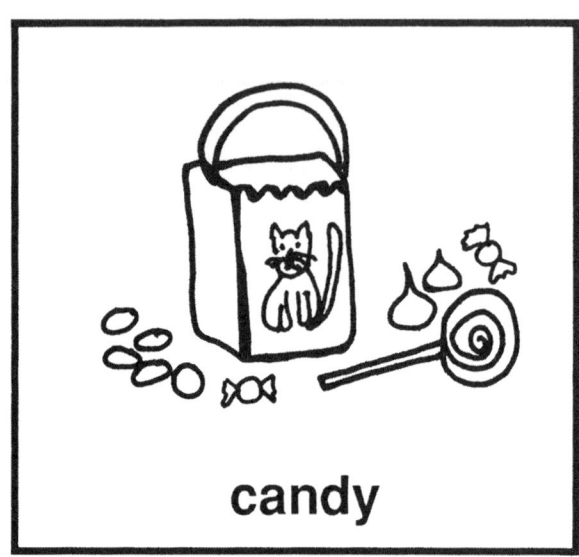

candy

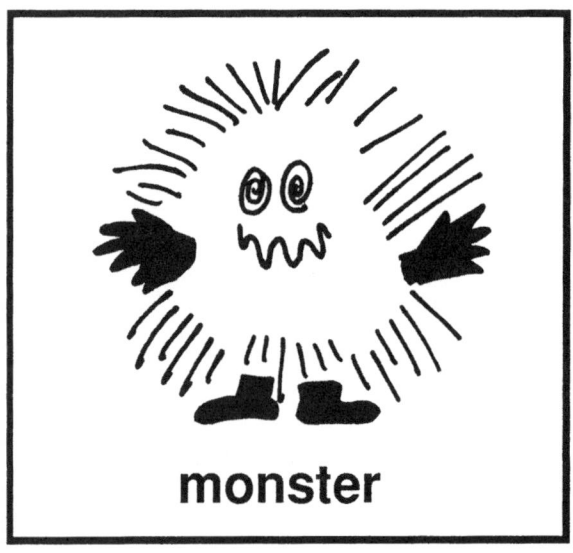

monster

costume

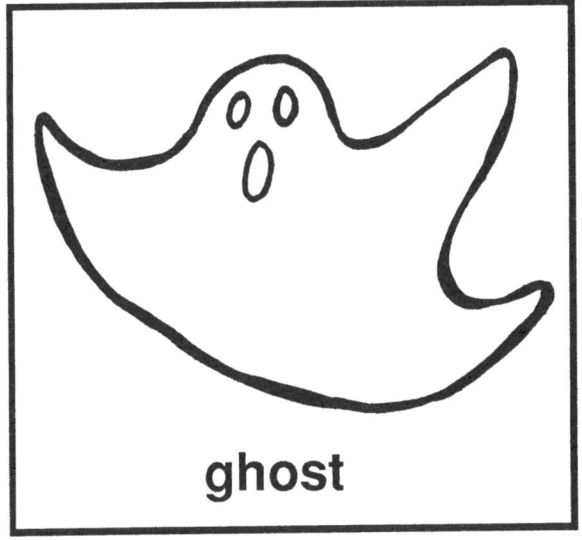

ghost

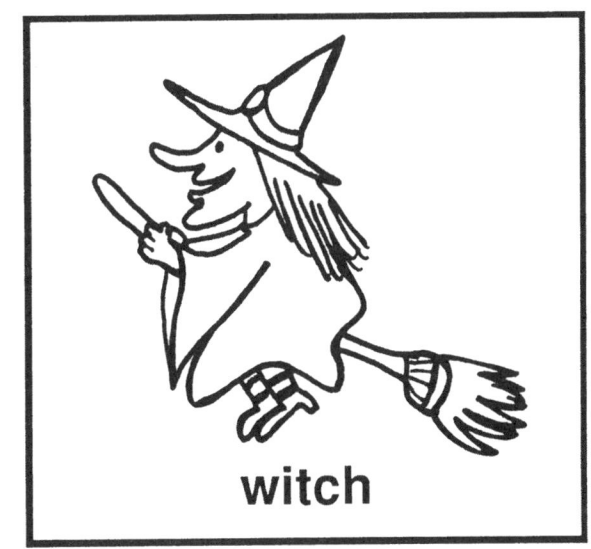

witch

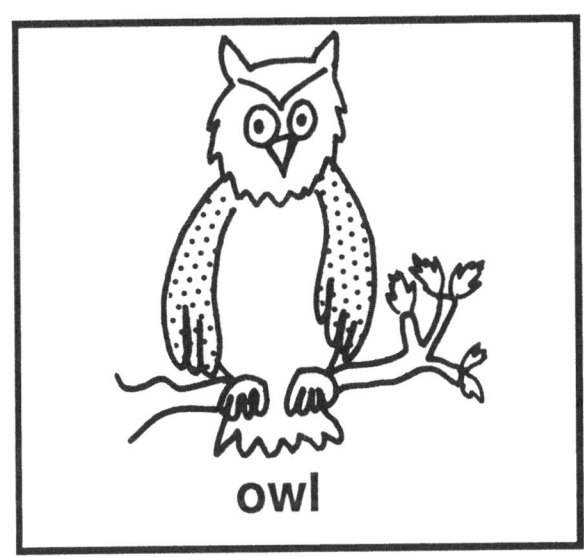

owl

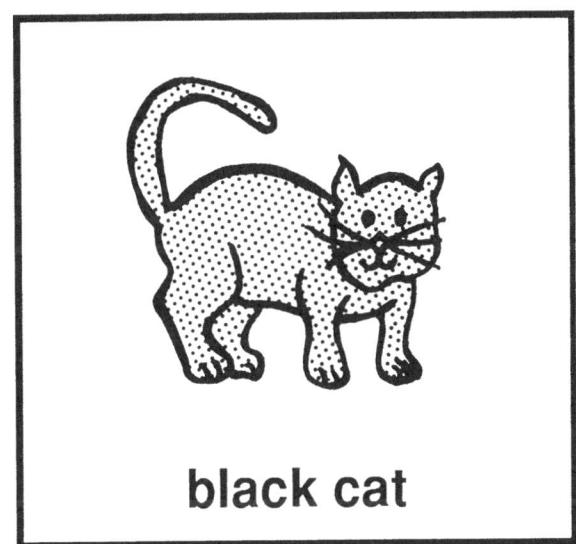

black cat

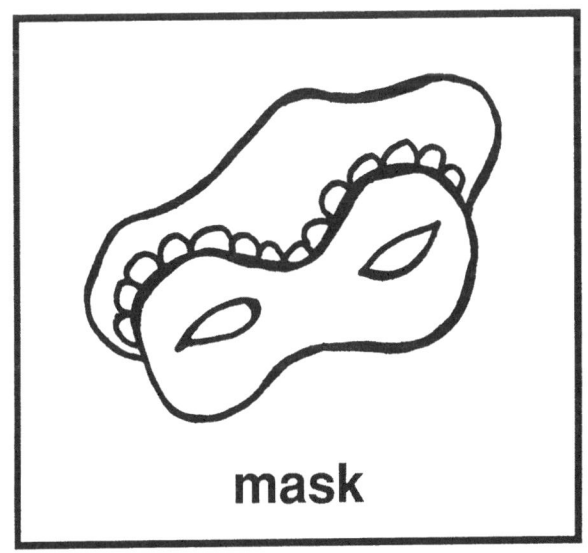

mask

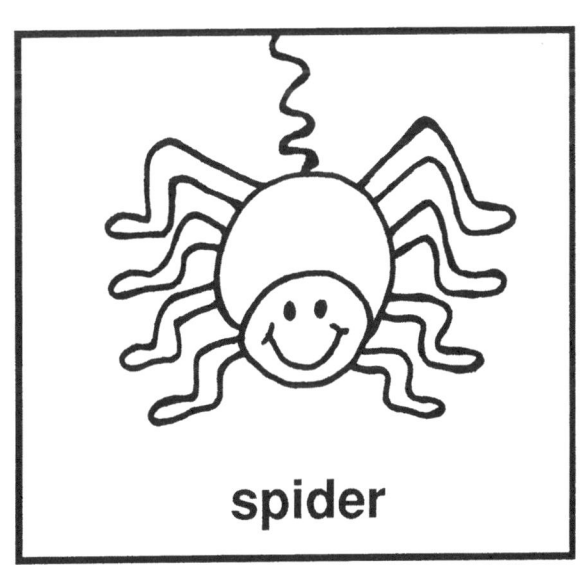

spider

3

Riddle Time

Instructor: Read each riddle below. Have the child choose which picture is being described. When the child chooses correctly, the picture can be colored.

1. It is an animal.
   It is black.
   It has wings.
   It flies.
   It is furry.
   It eats insects.
   What is it? (bat)

2. It is a Halloween creature.
   It is white.
   It says, "Boo!"
   What is it? (ghost)

3. It is a Halloween creature.
   It is ugly.
   It wears a big black hat.
   It rides on a broom.
   It says, "Heh, heh, heh."
   What is it? (witch)

4. It is an animal.
   It is black.
   It has whiskers.
   It has a long tail.
   It is furry.
   It says, "Meow."
   What is it? (cat)

5. It is something you wear.
   You wear it on Halloween.
   It can be funny or scary.
   You wear it on your face.
   What is it? (mask)

6. It is an animal.
   It has feathers.
   It has a beak.
   It flies.
   It says, "Who-o-o."
   What is it? (owl)

7. It is something you wear.
   You wear it on Halloween.
   It can be scary or funny.
   It is made of cloth or plastic.
   It can look like a witch, clown,
     or ghost.
   What is it? (costume)

8. It is made from a pumpkin.
   It is round and orange.
   It has two eyes, a nose ,
     and mouth.
   You make it on Halloween.
   You can put a candle inside.
   What is it? (jack-o-lantern)

9. It is something to eat.
   It tastes sweet.
   People put it in your
     "trick or treat" bag.
   To get it you say,
     "trick or treat."
   What is it? (candy)

10. It is a Halloween creature.
    It is big.
    It is ugly.
    It can be green, purple,
      or any color.
    It says, "Ar-r-r-g."
    What is it? (monster)

11. It is an animal.
    It is an insect.
    It crawls.
    It makes a web.
    It has 8 legs.
    What is it? (spider)

12. It is a Halloween creature.
    It is made of bones.
    It is white.
    It has arms and legs.
    What is it? (skeleton)

Other Suggestions/Activities

- Have the child name each picture and color it.

- Have the child choose a picture and describe it or have the child make up his own riddle.

- Say a sentence and have the child listen for a key word; i.e. "A <u>bat</u> flew over the moon." When the child hears the word <u>bat,</u> he draws a circle around the <u>bat.</u>

Riddle Time

Halloween - Worksheet 2

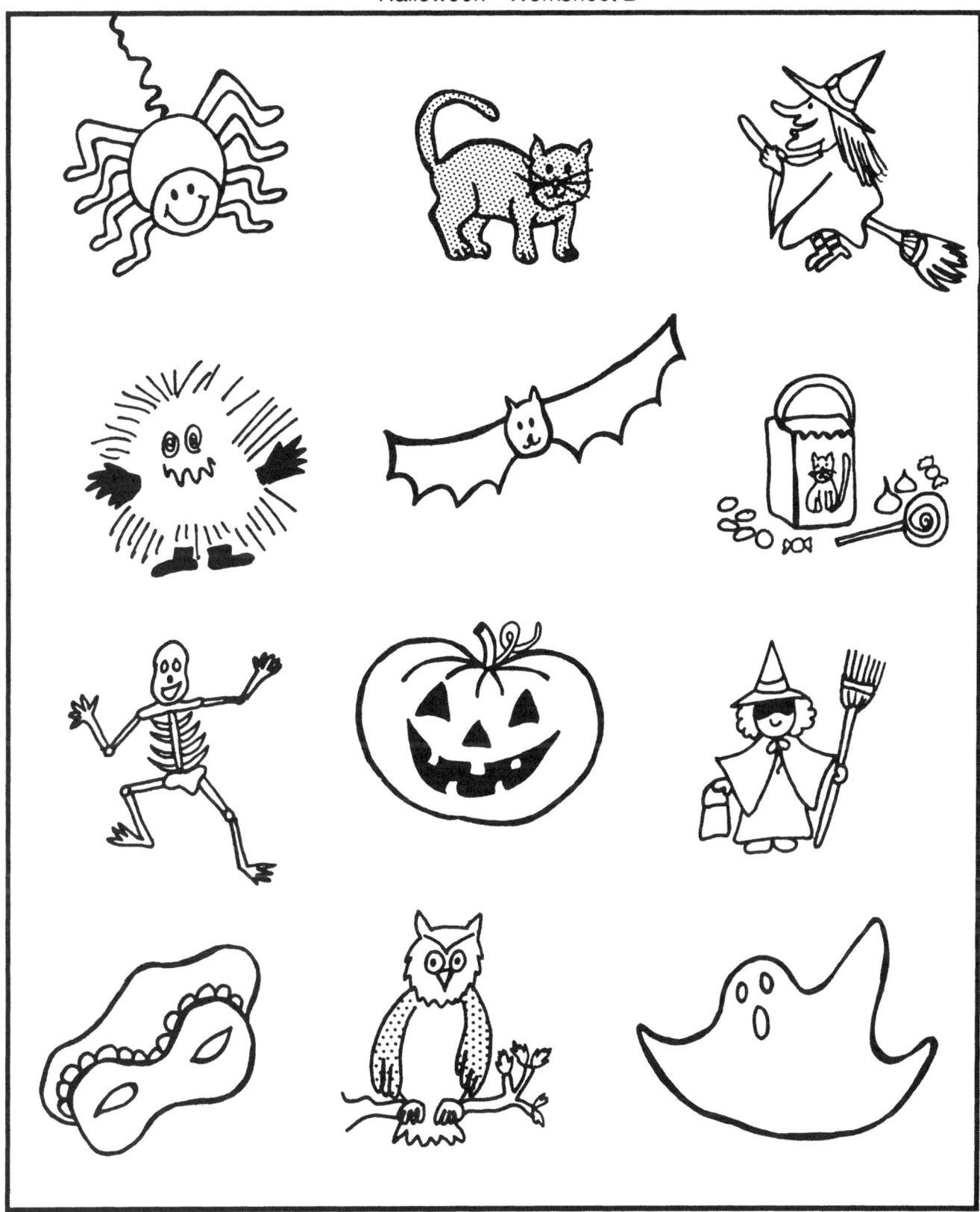

Name _____ Date _____

Spin a Word

<u>Instructor</u>: Have the child color and cut out spinner. Paste on heavy cardboard. Use a brad to connect the spinner.

Listen and Say

<u>Instructor</u>: "After you spin, I will ask you a question about your word."

1.	(ghost)	What does a ghost say?
2.	(monster)	What does a monster do?
3.	(candy)	How do you get candy in your trick-or-treat bag?
4.	(cat)	How does a black cat feel?
5.	(mask)	Where do you wear a mask?
6.	(spider)	How many legs does a spider have?
7.	(jack-o-lantern)	What can you put inside of a jack-o-lantern?
8.	(bat)	What does a bat eat?
9.	(witch)	What does a witch ride?
10.	(skeleton)	What is a skeleton made of?
11.	(owl)	Where does an owl live?
12.	(costume)	What kind of costume do you wear on Halloween?

Other Suggestions/Activities

- The child spins and tells about the picture.

> Ex: It is an owl.
> An owl is a bird.
> It has feathers.
> It says, "Who-o-o!"

- The child spins and gives a description of his picture not giving the name. The other children guess what picture is being described.

- The child spins and uses the word in a short sentence.

6

Spin a Word

Halloween - Worksheet 3

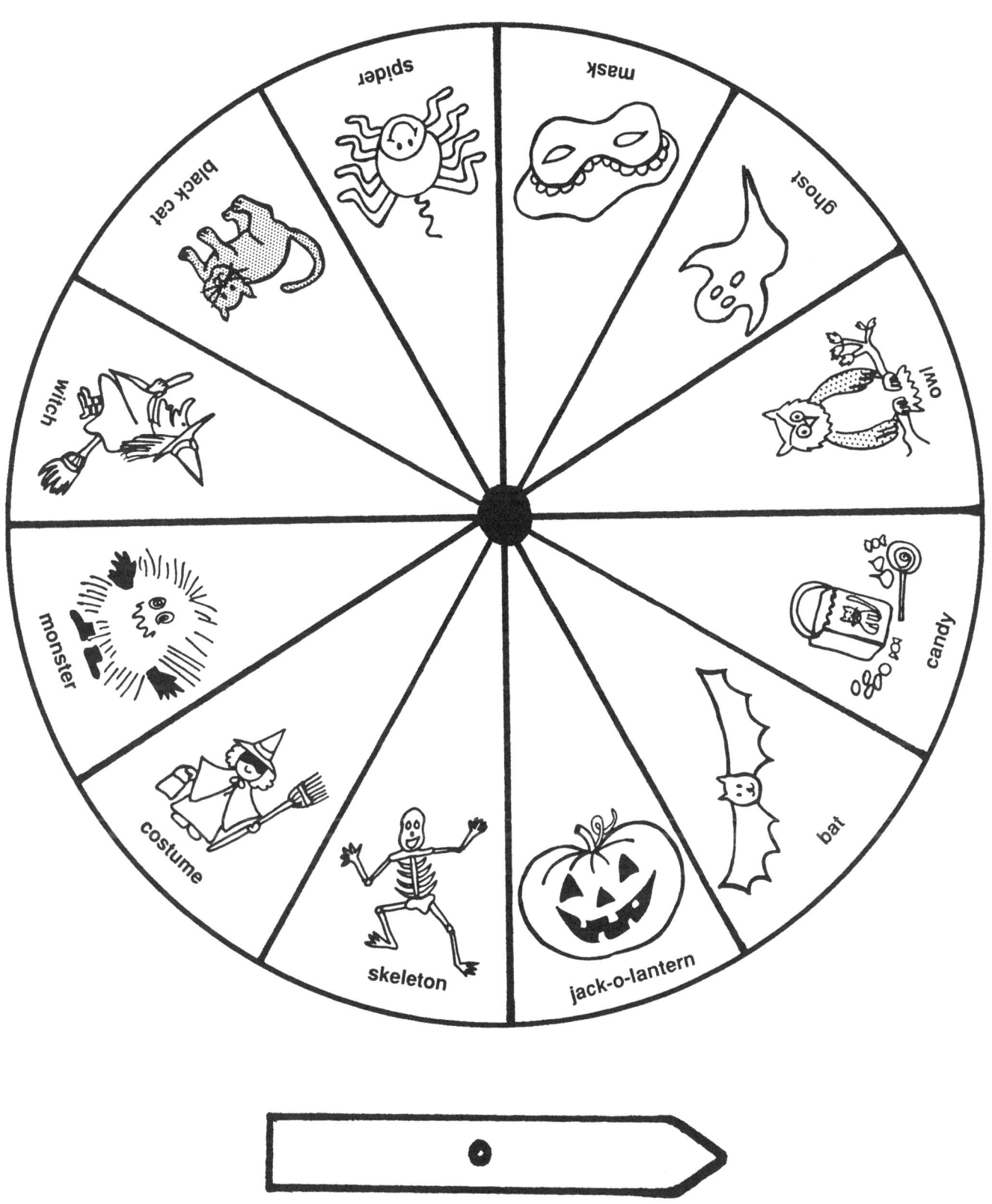

Who is Hiding?
Halloween - Worksheet 4

Yes/No Questions

Instructor: "Listen carefully. I will tell you something. If I am right, answer yes. If I am wrong, answer no." (When the child's response is correct, a part of the picture can be colored.)

1. The owl says, "Who-o-o." (yes)
2. Jack-o-lanterns are made from apples. (no)
3. Children wear costumes on Halloween. (yes)
4. Bats can fly. (yes)
5. Monsters scare people. (yes)
6. Witches wear black hats. (yes)
7. Children wear masks on their feet. (no)
8. Candy tastes sweet. (yes)
9. A cat has whiskers. (yes)
10. A spider has two legs. (no)
11. A skeleton is made from bones. (yes)
12. A ghost says "Meow." (no)

Sentence Completion

Instructor: "Listen carefully. I will say part of a sentence. When I stop, you say a word to finish the sentence." (When the child's response is correct, a part of the picture can be colored.)

1. A bat catches _____. (insects)
2. A ghost says _____. (boo)
3. A witch rides on a _____. (broom)
4. A cat says _____. (meow)
5. You wear a mask on your _____. (face)
6. An owl says _____. (Who-o-o)
7. A costume can be scary or _____. (funny)
8. A jack-o-lantern is made from a _____. (pumpkin)
9. People put candy in your trick-or-treat _____. (bag)
10. A monster says _____. (Ar-r-r-g)
11. A spider has eight _____. (legs)
12. A skeleton is made from _____. (bones)

Other Suggestion/Activities

- Read the child a book about bats. Discuss and ask questions (i.e. Can a bat fly?).

- Have the chlild color the page and hang on the bulletin board.

8

Who is Hiding?

Color the B spaces black and the O spaces orange.
What do you see?

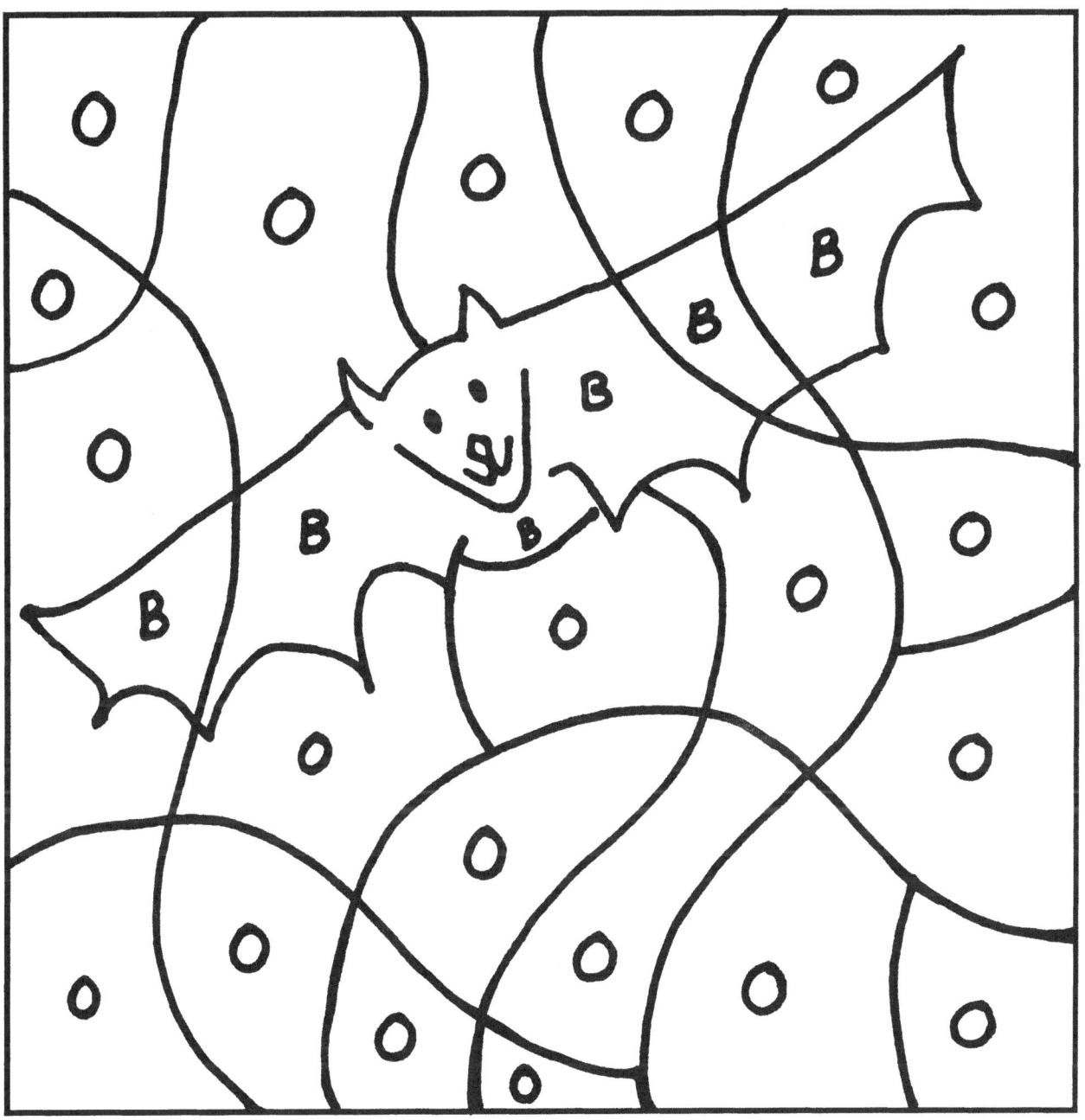

Name _____ Date _____

Let's Listen

Instructor: Discuss "big and little" and talk about the pictures.

Listen and Do

Instructor: Have child listen and follow directions. "Listen carefully and do what I say."

1. Draw a line from the big cat to the little cat.
2. Color the big cat black.
3. Draw a line from the big ghost to the little ghost.
4. Color the big ghost white.
5. Draw a line from the big pumpkin to the little pumpkin.
6. Color the little pumpkin orange.
7. Draw a line from the big bat to the little bat.
8. Color the big bat black.
9. Draw a line from the big owl to the little owl.
10. Color the little owl brown.
11. Color the big owl black.
12. Color the little bat orange.
13. Color the little ghost green.
14. Color the little cat orange.
15. Color the big pumpkin orange.

Other Suggestions/Activities

- Use for two step directions. Ex: Color the big cat black and the little cat orange.

- Color and cut out pictures. Make big and little cards. Match big cat to little cat, or use for sorting - all big or all little.

- Use for the development of position words. (i.e. Draw a line <u>under</u> the big cat. Draw a line <u>over</u> the little cat.)

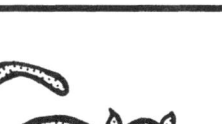

Listening

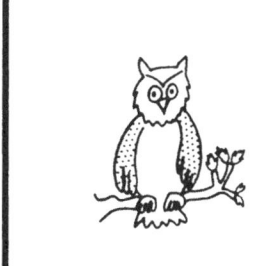

Halloween - Worksheet 5

big   little

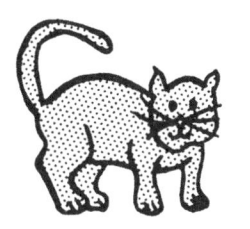
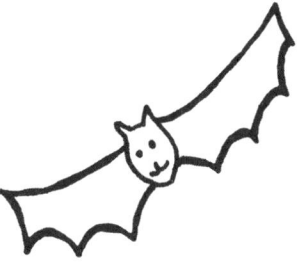

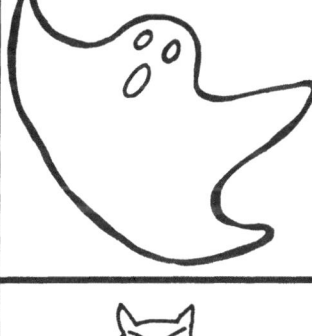
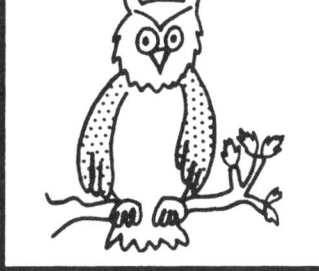

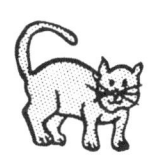
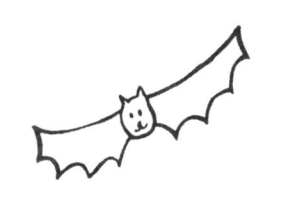
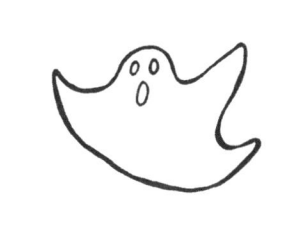

Name _____ Date _____

11

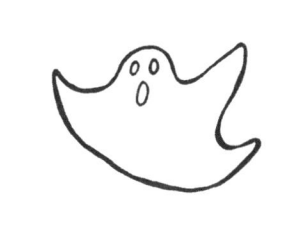

Following Directions

Visual Discrimination - Motor Activity

Instructor: Have the child examine each picture individually. Have the child tell you what is missing. If the child needs help getting started, try the following:

Ex: "A witch usually flies on a broom. Look carefully at this witch. Is anything missing?"

After the child tells you what is missing from each picture have him draw the missing items on the pictures.

Auditory Discrimination

Instructor: "Listen carefully and do as I say."

"Draw a tail on the cat."
"Draw a broom for the witch."
"Draw eyes on the pumpkin."
"Draw a mouth and eyes on the ghost."
"Draw legs on the spider."
"Draw eyes on the monster."

Other Suggestions/Activities

- Use for the development of basic concept words: i.e. "Draw a line under the witch, draw a square over the ghost."

- Use for "I am Thinking" game. The instructor says, "I am thinking of an animal. It has whiskers, a long tail, and is furry. What is it?"

Following Directions

Halloween - Worksheet 6

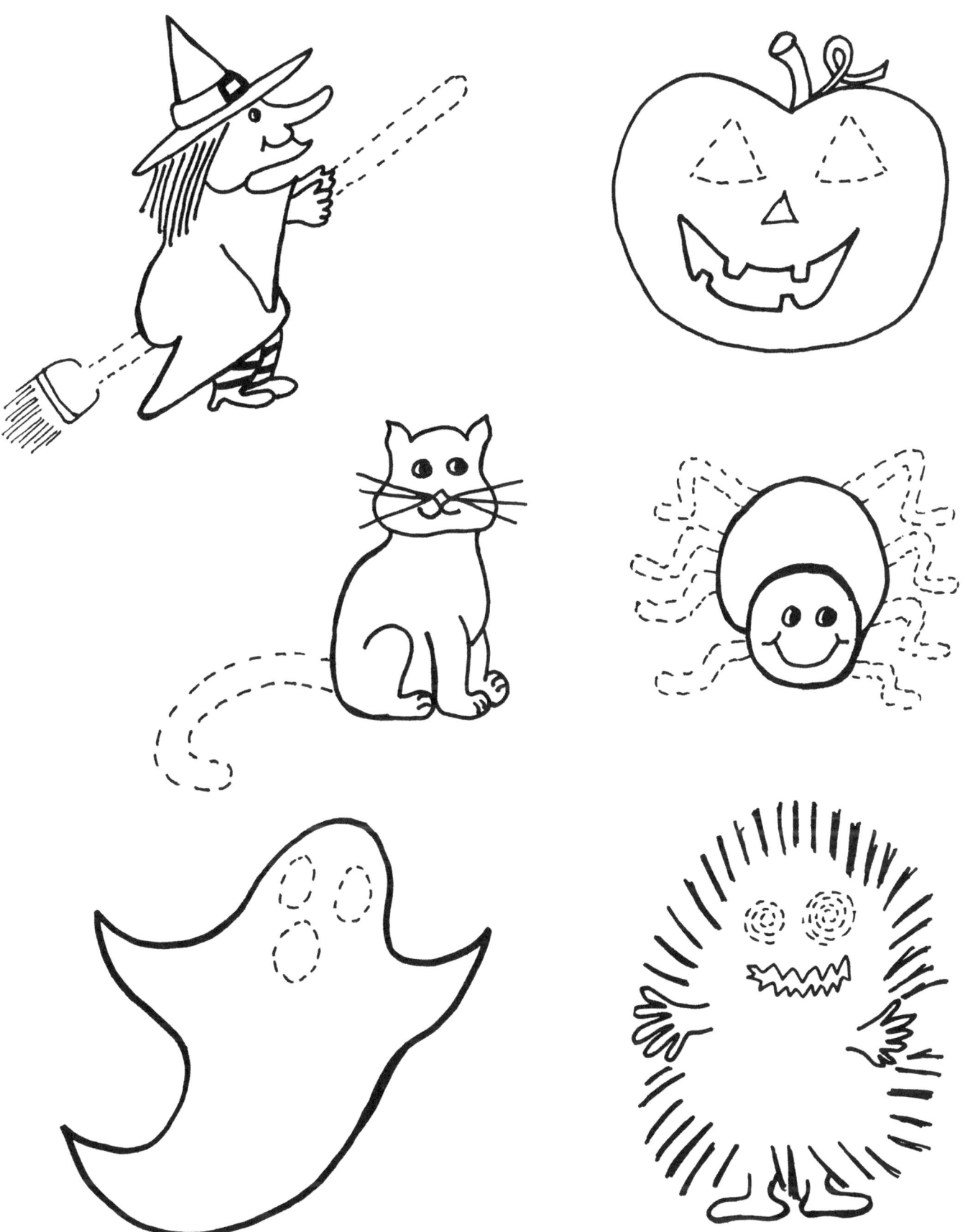

13

Pumpkin Time

Instructor: Discuss how pumpkins grow.

> Ex: Pumpkins grow from seeds. They are fruits. The plant makes a vine and the pumpkins grow there. A small place where pumpkins grow can be called a pumpkin patch.

Sequence Activity

Have child color and cut out each picture. The child can put the pictures in order and paste on a piece of construction paper.

Listen and Say

Instructor: This activity allows child to listen to a question and then immediately respond. Read the statement then ask the child the question.

1. Pumpkins have a round shape.
   What shape are pumpkins?

2. Pumpkins grow on vines.
   Where do pumpkins grow?

3. Jack-o-lanterns are made from pumpkins.
   What are jack-o-lanterns made from?

4. We scrape seeds out of a pumpkin.
   What do we scrape out of a pumpkin?

5. We make two eyes on a pumpkin.
   How many eyes do we make?

Other Suggestions/Activities

- Discuss how a pumpkin is made into a jack-o-lantern.

- Bring a pumpkin to class. Have the child help make a jack-o-lantern.

Pumpkin Time

Halloween - Worksheet 7

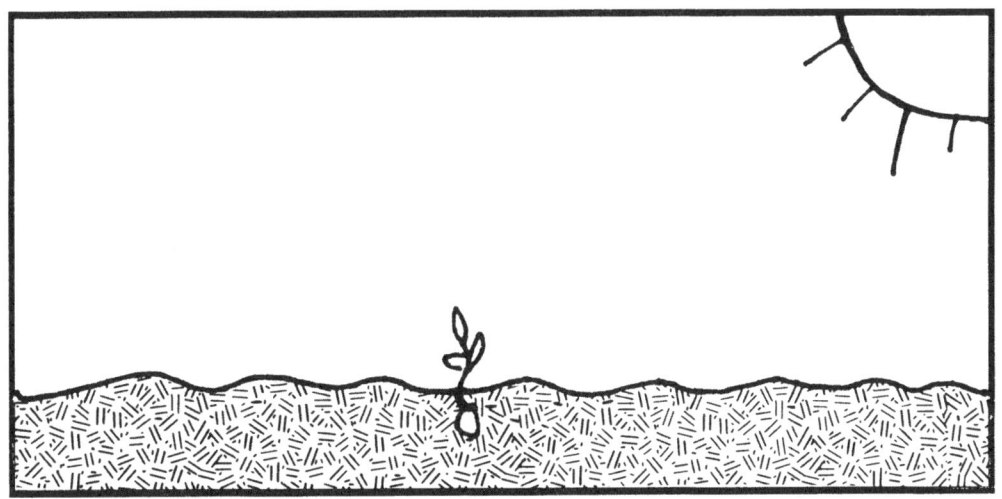

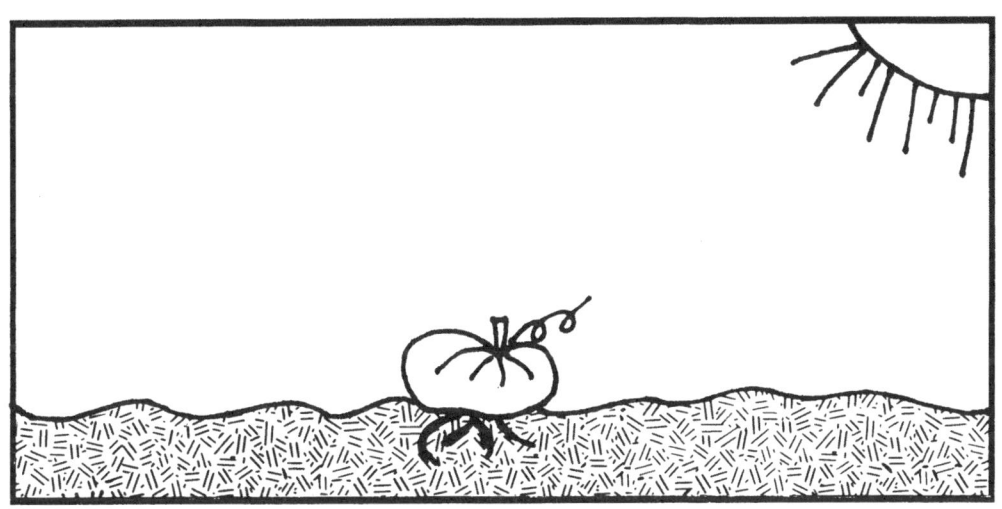

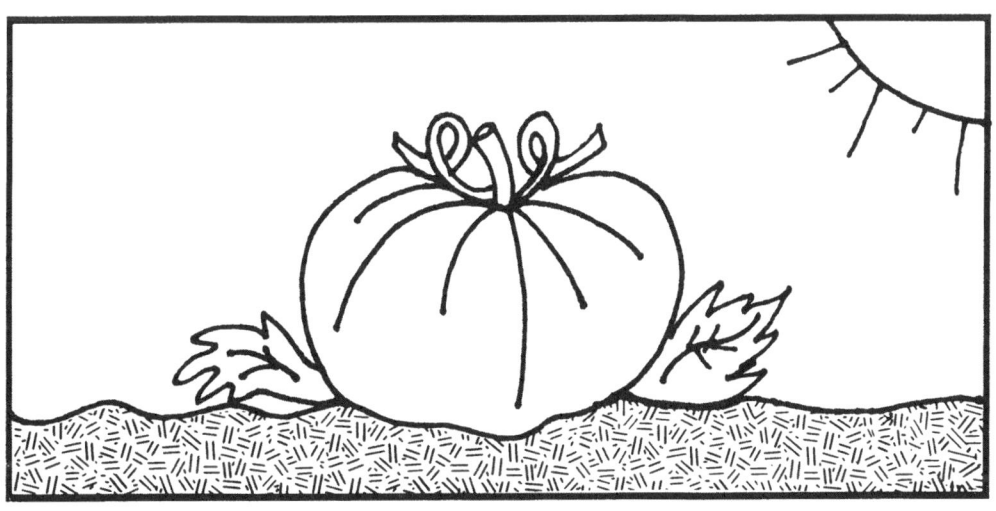

15

Five Little Pumpkins

Halloween - Worksheet 8

Instructor: Have child color and cut out pumpkins. Read Five Little Pumpkins poem below. As you say each verse, have child paste a pumpkin on his pumpkin patch.

Five Little Pumpkins

One little pumpkin, growing on a vine.
The little pumpkin said, "This patch is mine!"

Two little pumpkins, sitting on the ground,
"My we're growing big and orange and round."

Three little pumpkins, happy in the sun,
Then one said, "Having friends is fun."

Four little pumpkins - they all let out a roar,
"We only have room for just one more!"

Five little pumpkins, smiling big and bright,
They all said together, "This is just right."

Other Suggestions/Activities

- As child can repeat each verse of the poem, a pumpkin can be pasted on the pumpkin patch.

- Number the pumpkins 1-5. Have the child practice counting his pumpkins in his pumpkin patch.

- Use poem with stick puppets made from pumpkins on page 17. Have child learn poem and recite it. This activity can be used with a group of four or five children. Have each child memorize one verse of the poem.

Five Little Pumpkins

Halloween - Worksheet 8

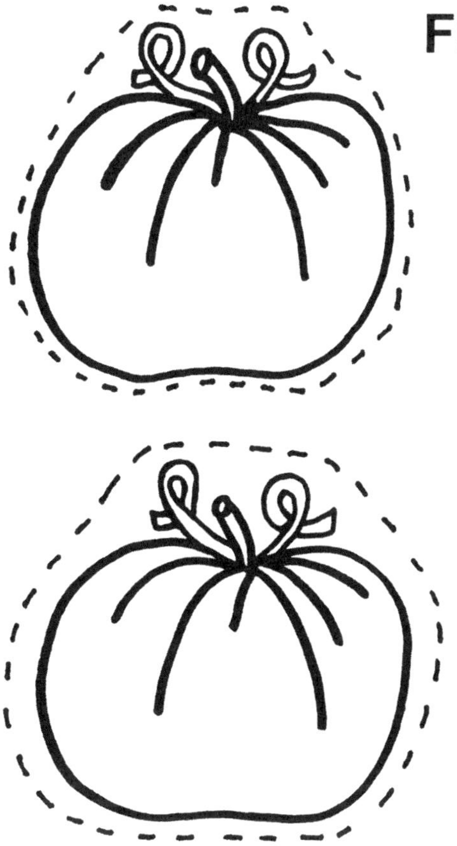

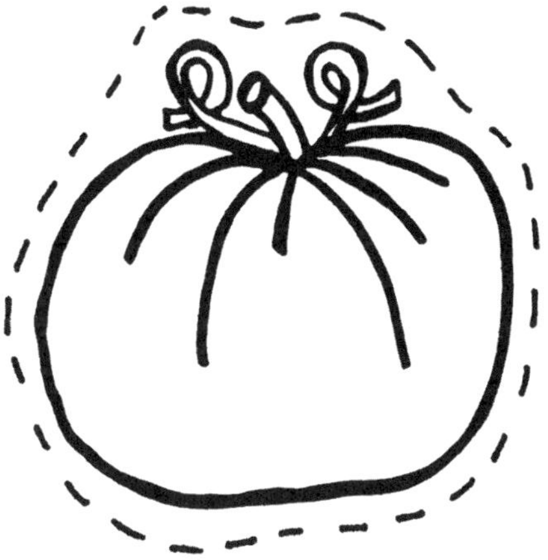

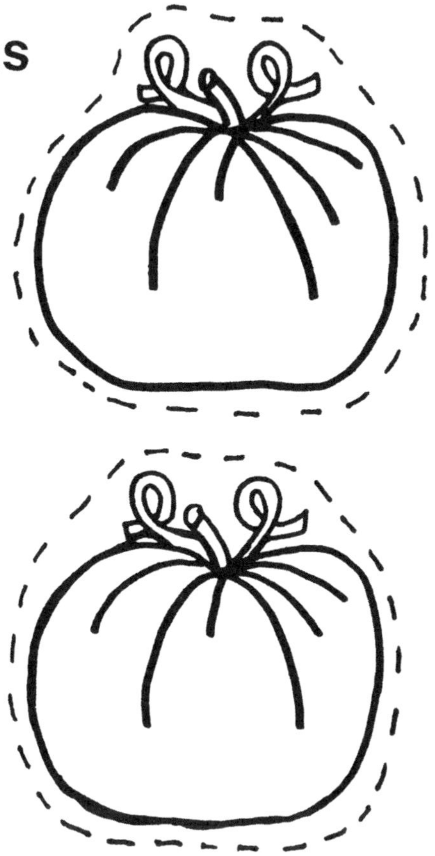

My Pumpkin Patch

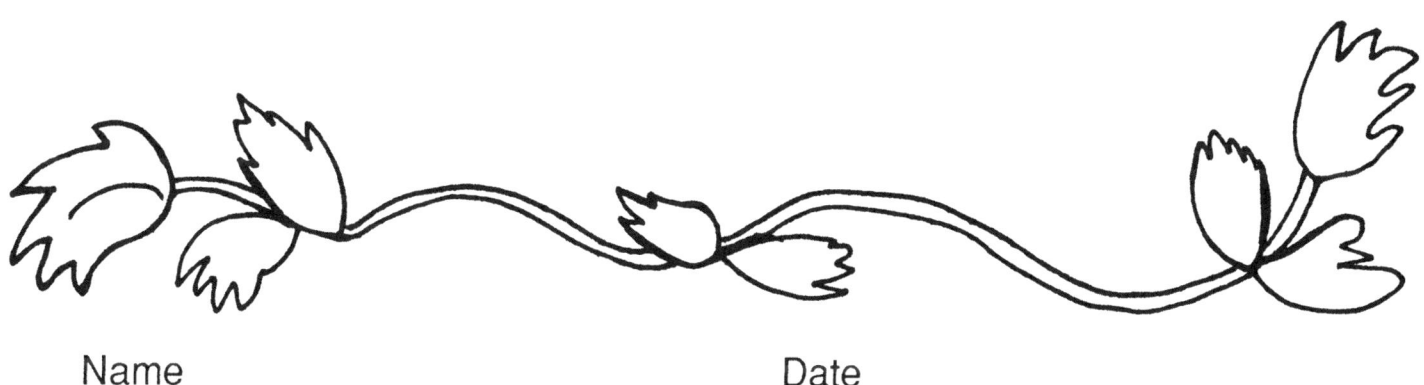

Name ______________________________ Date ______________________________

Rhyming Time

<u>Instructor</u>: Reproduce stick puppets on page 19. Have the child color and cut out.
Paste each character to the end of a tongue depressor or popsicle stick.

Read a poem. Have the child hold up a stick puppet when he hears the
name of his character.

<u>Poem Time</u>

Halloween

The owl says Who-o-o-o,
The ghost says Boo!
I'm not afraid---
Are you?

The Witch and the Bat

The witch has a hat,
It's very big and black,
It's grabbed by the bat
Who won't give it back.

Jack-o-lantern

The jack-o-lantern smiled at me,
His smile was very bright;
Jack-o-lantern can't you see,
I'm trick-or-treating tonight?

<u>Other Suggestion/Activities</u>

- Sentence completion: Read a poem and leave off the last word in a line. Have the
  child complete the line by saying the word.

- Have the child learn one poem and recite it using a stick puppet.

- Have the child recite a poem wearing a mask (page 25) made like a character in
  the poem.

- Rewrite a poem on large chart paper. Have the child draw a picture to go with the
  poem. Place on bulletin board.

Rhyming Time - Stick Puppets

Halloween - Worksheet 9

Instructions: Have child color then cut out each character. Paste each character to the end of a tongue depressor or popsicle stick.

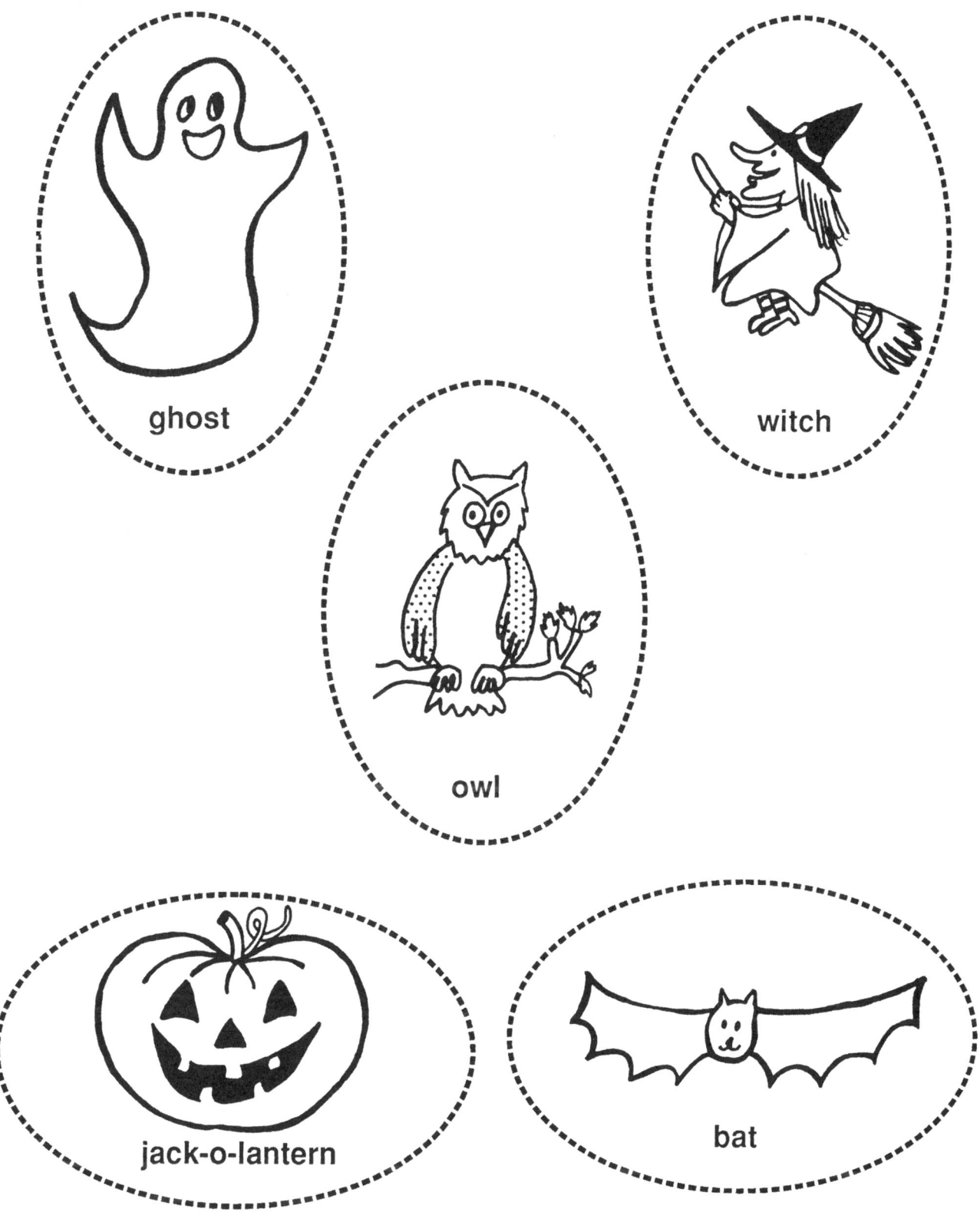

ghost

witch

owl

jack-o-lantern

bat

19

Halloween Story

Instructor: Read "A Halloween for Curtis" to the child. If possible, use props to assist in attending skills. (Have a pumpkin or jack-o-lantern nearby, dress up like a witch, wear a mask or special hat.)

Storytime

Reproduce stick puppets (page 23). Have the child color, cut out, and paste on a tongue depressor or popsicle stick. Use while telling the story or have children hold up a stick puppet when they hear the name of their character in the story.

Other Suggestions/Activities

- Read one paragraph at a time and ask "WH" questions.

       Ex: Paragraph 1
          Where did Curtis go?
          Who did he go with?
          What color were the leaves?

- Have the child draw a picture about the story and tell about his picture.

A Halloween for Curtis

Characters: Curtis, Mother, Father, Nicole, Kevin, Black cat, Monster, Witch

Curtis is going to the grocery store with his mother. It is a cool Fall day. The leaves are changing colors. Some are red. Others are yellow. It is a pretty day.

"We need to buy a pumpkin," says Mother. "Tonight is Halloween." "I want a big, orange, round pumpkin, " says Curtis. "We can make a jack-o-lantern." Curtis sees a big, orange, round pumpkin in the grocery store. "I bet this one was the biggest one on the vine."

When Curtis gets home he shows the pumpkin to his father. "Let's make a jack-o-lantern right now," says Curtis. "Let's think and plan," says Father. "First, we draw a face on the pumpkin. We can draw two triangles for eyes and one for the nose. We draw a big smile for the mouth. Second, we cut out the top of the pumpkin around the green stem. We take the top off and scrape out all the seeds. We cut out his face - - eyes, nose, and big smile. Last, we put a candle inside. We can light the candle at night so the pumpkin can glow."

Curtis and his father make a very funny jack-o-lantern from their pumpkin. "My jack-o-lantern is the biggest and best ever," says Curtis. Mother says, "Let's bake the pumpkin seeds for a snack. I'll make some pumpkin cookies, too." "Let me help," says Curtis. "I love to cook and I love to eat."

Curtis is playing in the yard and sees Kevin, his friend. "Tonight is Halloween. We need a costume," says Curtis. "I want to dress up in a scary costume. I want to be a monster." Kevin thinks for a minute and says, "I want to wear a black cat costume. People are afraid of black cats. They have green eyes that glow in the dark." "Yes," says Curtis, "black cats are always with ugly witches. My sister, Nicole, is going to be a witch. She has a big black hat to wear and a big broom to ride."

"Dad is taking us trick or treating," says Curtis. "We will see lots of costumes." Some people dress up like skeletons, tigers, pumpkins,

21

clowns, and ghosts. We'll see all kinds of wild creatures," says Kevin. "Halloween is so much fun," says Curtis. "I like to say 'trick or treat' at each house and get candy in my bag."

That night a witch, black cat, and monster are ready for a big night of treats. Dad says, "Remember kids -- safety is important. What do we need to remember?" Curtis says, "All candy should be wrapped. We don't eat it until you check it." Kevin says, "I know -- we stay in groups. We go to houses we know. Nicole says, "We use a flashlight to see at night. We never, never, get in a car with a stranger." "You kids are great," says Mom. "Have fun and remember to be careful."

Dad takes the three creatures around the neighborhood. They hear scary sounds -- an owl who says 'who-o-o-o' and a ghost who says 'boo!' They see many scary costumes. The three scariest are the monster, witch, and black cat. They go to each door and say, "trick or treat." They get lots of candy and gum. They also get pencils, spider rings, and other great treats.

When they come home, Mom checks all the things in the bags. "You really have the loot," says Mom . Dad says, "There is a big haunted house with many scary things near the mall. Do you creatures want to go?" "A-r-r-r-r-g," says the monster, "Meow," says the cat, and the witch jumps on her broom.

Halloween Story - Stick Puppets

Halloween - Worksheet 10

Instructions: Have child color then cut out each character. Paste each character to the end of a tongue depressor or popsicle stick.

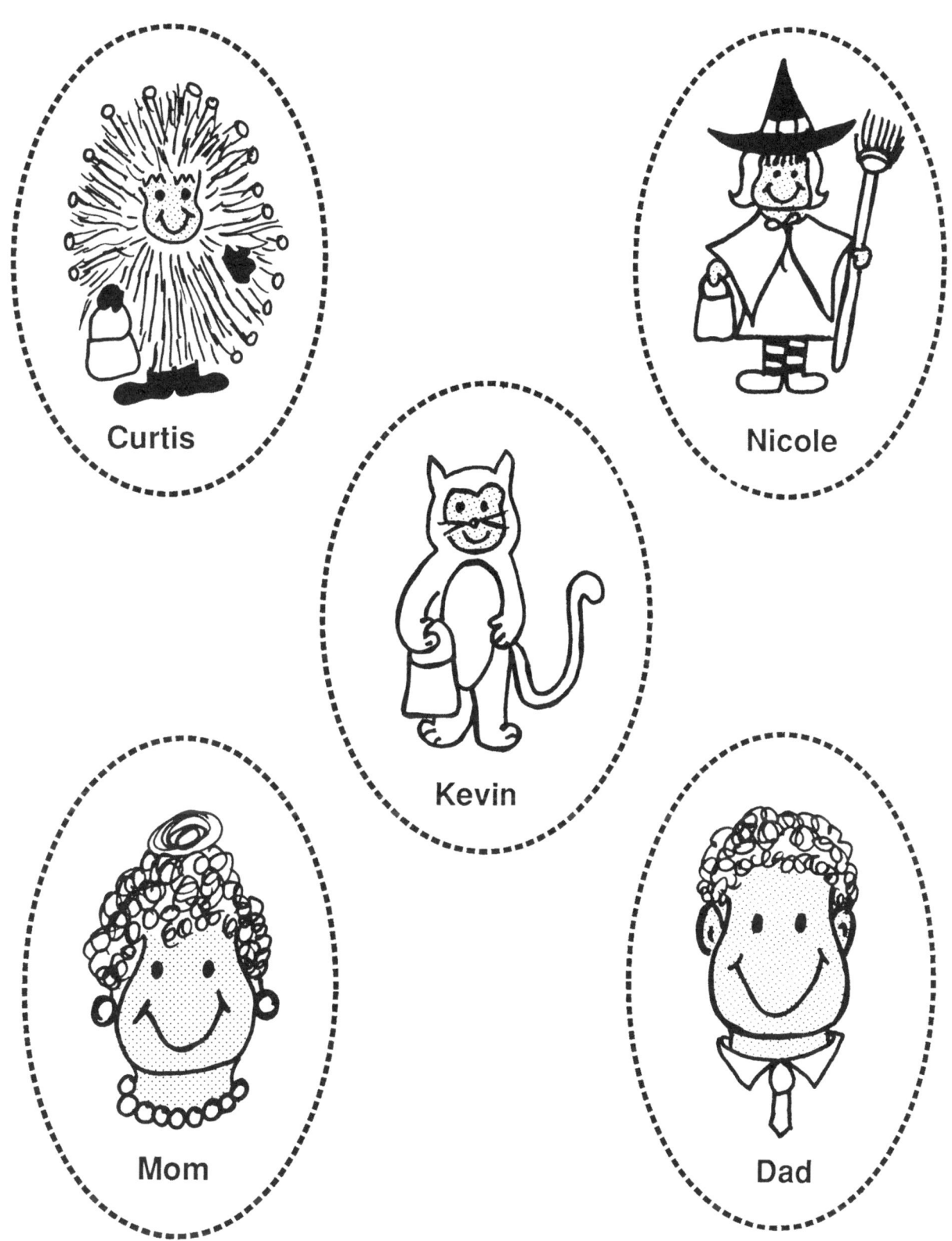

Curtis

Nicole

Kevin

Mom

Dad

23

A Halloween Play

Instructor: Have child create a mask for a Halloween character of his choice. The child can then act out or tell about his character.

Short Play

Instructor: Have children create a mask for an owl, witch, monster, ghost, and bat. Have children perform play.

WITCH: "I love Halloween. I like to scare people with my funny laugh. Heh, Heh, Heh!"

GHOST: "I like to jump out and say - Boo!"

BAT: "I like to fly around at night. That really scares people."

MONSTER: "People just look at me and run away."

OWL: "Who-o-o-o! (Everyone acts afraid and runs away.)

Other Suggestions/Activities

- Have child say a poem or riddle about his character.

Halloween Mask

Halloween - Worksheet 11

Instructions: Have the child create a mask for a Halloween character.   Paste mask on heavier paper for added durability. Now cut the mask out. Use string or yarn for tying.

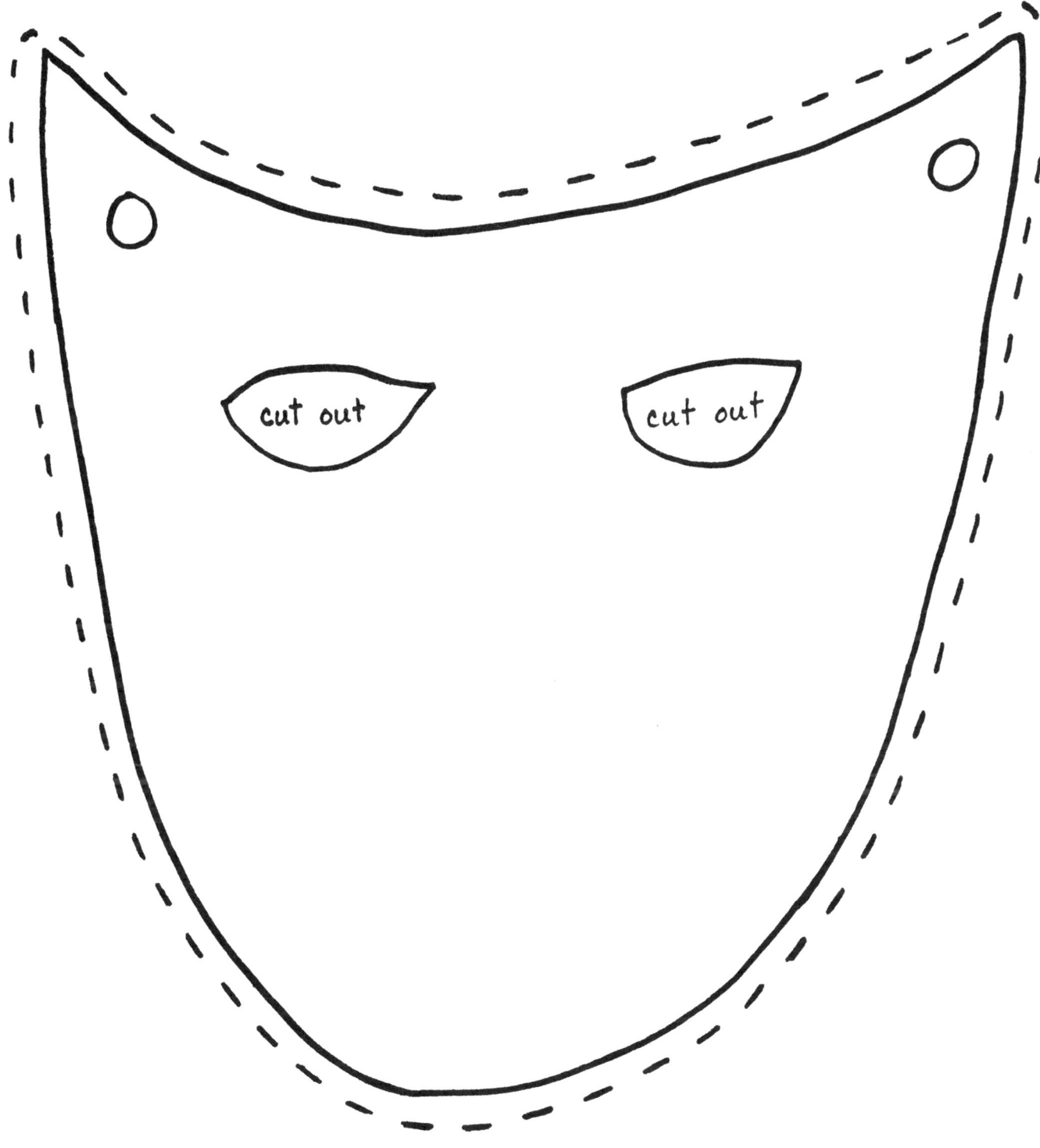

cut out

cut out

25

Halloween Game

Instructor: Each child selects a marker; i.e. button or pawn. Flipping a penny can be used to determine movement. Ex: Heads - move ahead one space, tails - move ahead two spaces.

Reproduce one set of picture cards (pages 2 and 3). Have the child name the picture or tell one thing about the picture before he moves.

Other Suggestions/Activities

- Use the game board for the development of other vocabulary. Ex: Colors, basic concept words, numbers.

- Use in conjunction with riddles (page 4), yes/no questions (page 8), or sentence completion (page 8). Have the child respond before moving.

- Use for unit review.

Can you help the witch get to her broom?

Caught in a spider web. Lose a turn.

Take an extra turn!

Witch says, "Go to pumpkin patch."

Pumpkin Patch

Scary ghost, go back one space.

Bat says, "Move ahead 2 spaces."

Saw a black cat. Lose a turn.

27

Let's Talk About Thanksgiving

Introduction to Thanksgiving

Instructor: Tell the child about Thanksgiving.

Ex: Thanksgiving is a holiday that we celebrate in November. It is on the 3rd Thursday in November. Thanksgiving began when the Pilgrims came to America. The Pilgrims made friends with the Indians. The Indians helped the Pilgrims plant their crops. When their crops were ready to harvest, they celebrated. They were ready for winter.

Animals and plants get ready for winter, too. Trees begin to lose their leaves. Animals begin to store food for winter.

Core Vocabulary

Use the picture cards (pages 30 and 31) to introduce the Thanksgiving core vocabulary. Have the child color the pictures. The pictures may be cut out and mounted on light cardboard. Describe each picture. Tell about the size, color, and particular attributes of each object.

Match-up Activity

Reproduce two of each picture to make a set. Have the child find the matching pictures after you scramble them.

Memory Game

Place two to four cards on the table. Have the child look at the cards for a few seconds. Cover or turn them over. Have the child name the pictures from memory.

Other Suggestions/Activities

- Have child categorize: plants, animals, people, food, non-living objects.

- Different/Alike. Place two pictures (i.e. corn - apple) on the table. Have the child tell you how they are different or how they are alike.

- Lay the cards on the table face up. Have the child listen to a sequence and follow the directions. Ex: Instructor say, "Pick up the hat, pie, and tree." Simplify the sequence or increase the difficulty as needed.

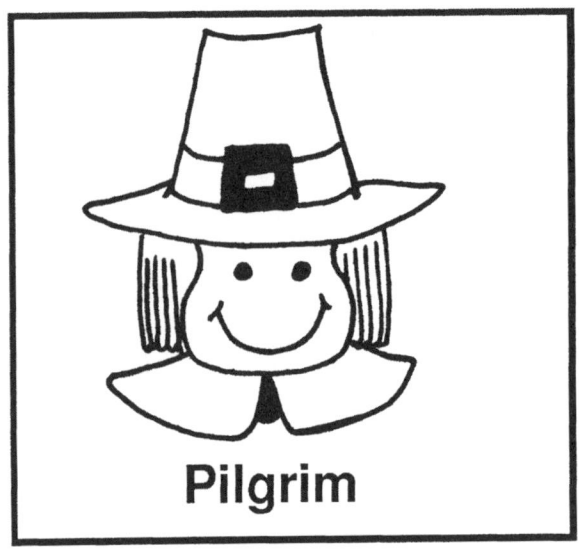

Pilgrim

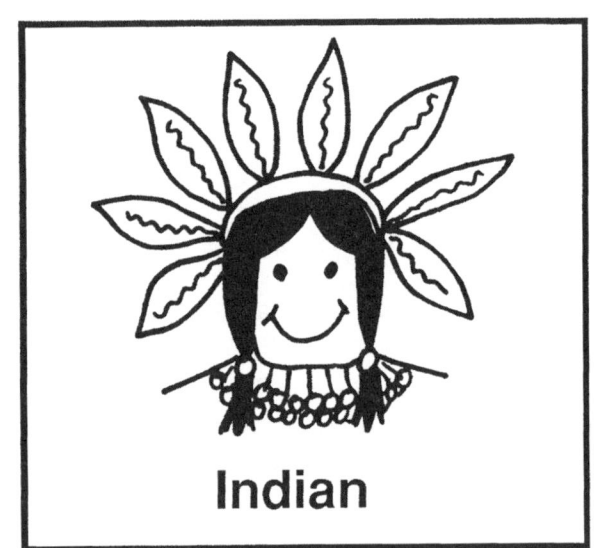

Indian

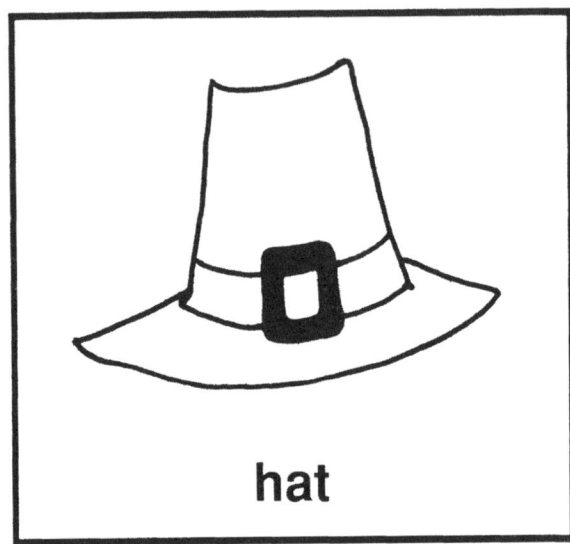

hat

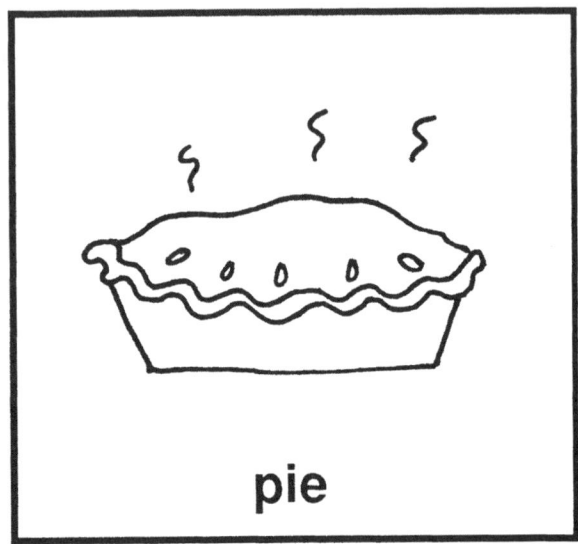

pie

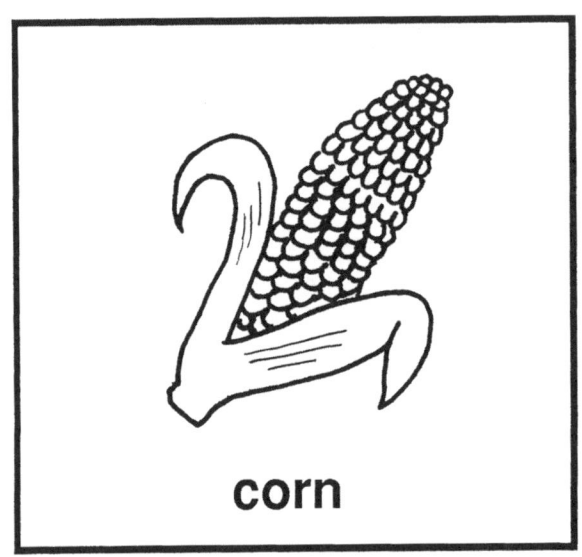

corn

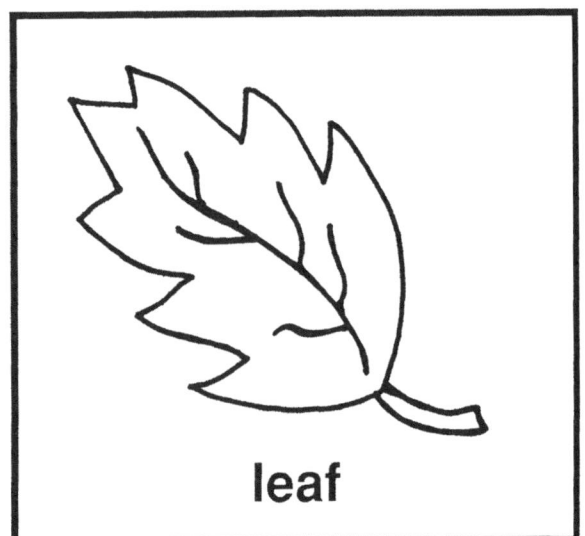

leaf

30

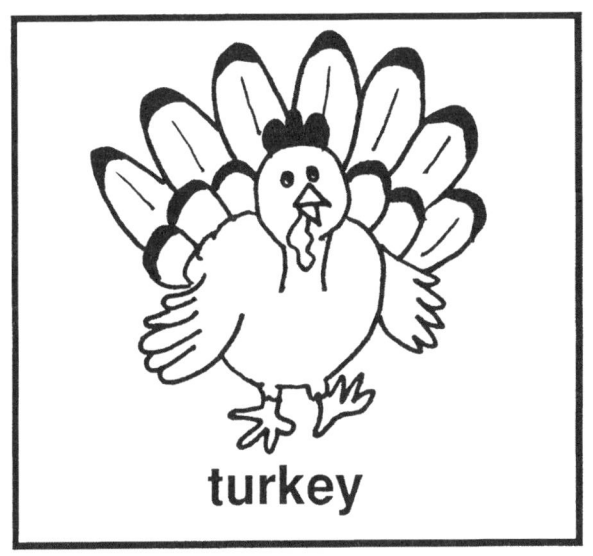

turkey

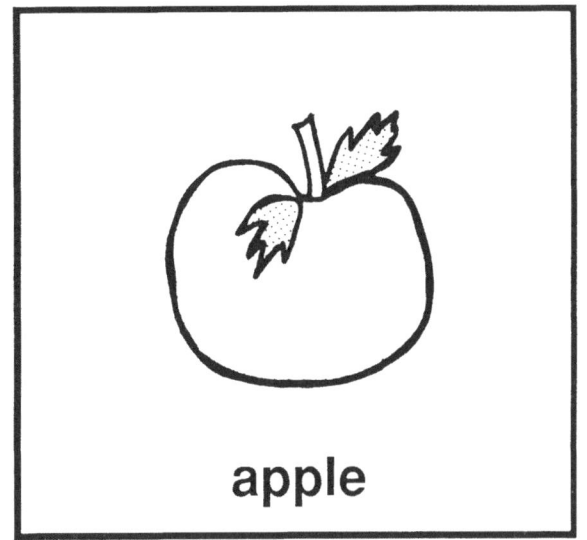

apple

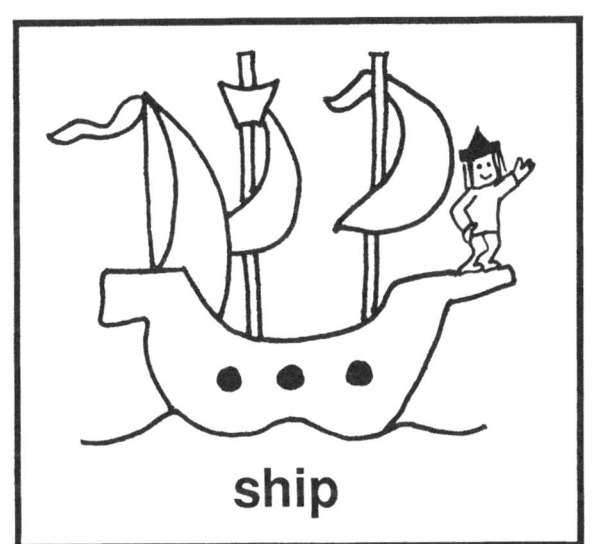

ship

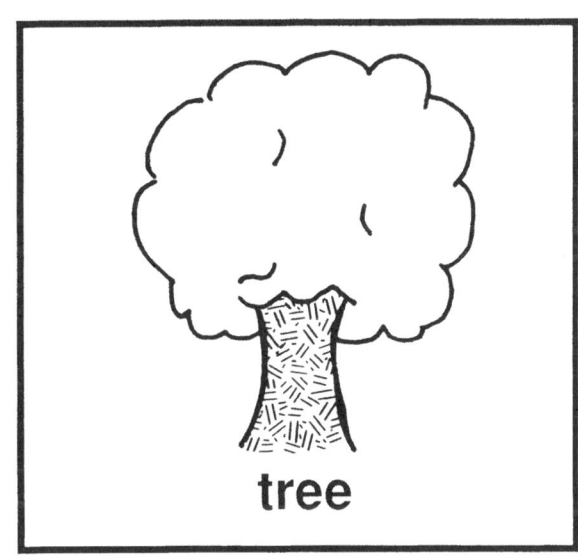

tree

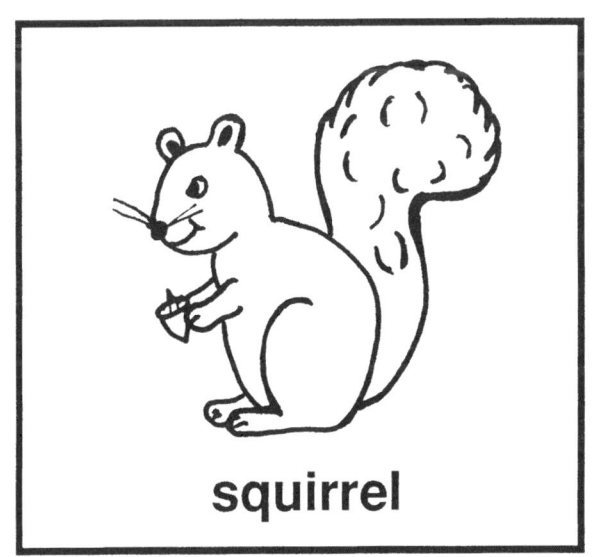

squirrel

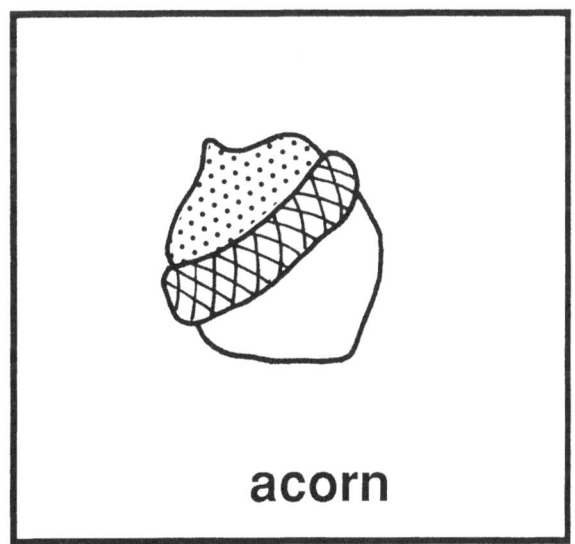

acorn

Riddle Time

Instructor: Read each riddle below. Have the child choose which picture is being described. When the child chooses correctly, the picture can be colored.

1. It is an animal.
   It is a bird.
   It has feathers.
   It goes "gobble, gobble."
   What is it? (turkey)

2. It travels on water.
   It is very big.
   It has sails.
   The Pilgrims came
     to America on this.
   What is it? (ship)

3. It is a food.
   It is a dessert.
   It is baked in the oven.
   It can be made from
     apples, pumpkin,
     or cherries.
   What is it? (pie)

4. It is a food.
   It is a vegetable.
   It has kernels.
   It grows on a tall stalk.
   What is it? (corn)

5. It is something to wear.
   You wear it on your head.
   It can keep your head warm
     or shade you from the sun.
   What is it? (hat)

6. It is a food.
   It is a fruit.
   It is red.
   It has a stem.
   When you bite into it,
     it goes "crunch."
   What is it? (apple)

7. It is a person.
   He wears a tall hat.
   He has a big white collar.
   He came to America on
     the Mayflower.
   Who is it? (Pilgrim)

8. It is little.
   It comes from an oak tree.
   Squirrels like them.
   What is it? (acorn)

9. It grows on a tree.
   It grows in spring.
   It falls off in autumn.
   It can change colors.
   It can be red, yellow,
     green, or brown.
   What is it? (leaf)

10. It is a person.
    He made friends with
      the Pilgrims.
    He helped the Pilgrims
      plant crops.
    Who is it? (Indian)

11. It is a plant.
    It has leaves.
    It has a trunk.
    It has branches.
    It is tall.
    What is it? (tree)

12. It is an animal.
    It is furry.
    It has a bushy tail.
    It climbs trees.
    It likes acorns.
    What is it? (squirrel)

Other Suggestions/Activities

- Use the Thanksgiving scene to talk about the first Thanksgiving celebrated by the Pilgrims and Indians.

- Have the child color the Thanksgiving scene and then tell a story about it.

- Have the child color and name all the objects in the scene.

Riddle Time

Thanksgiving - Worksheet 14

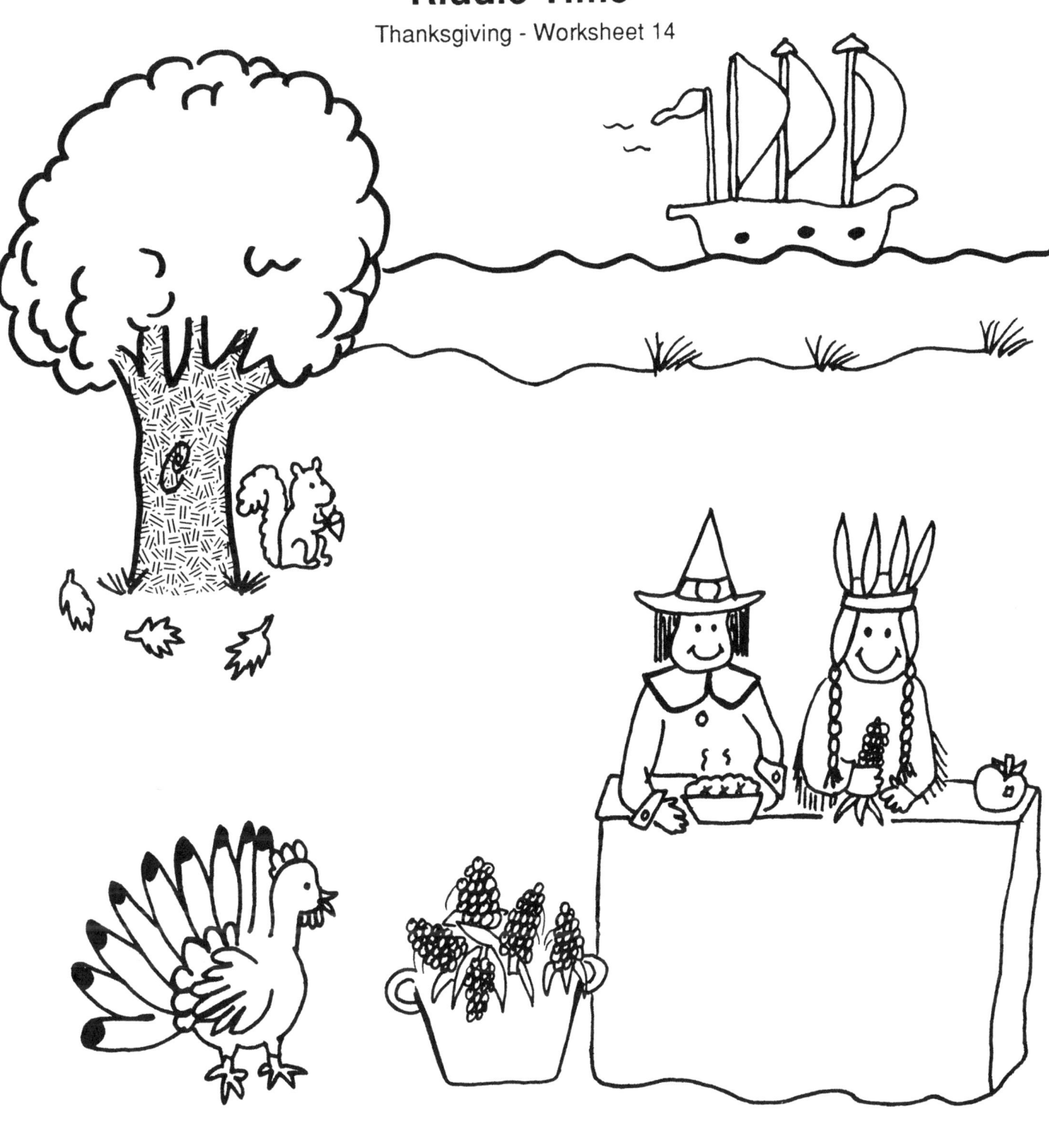

Name _____   Date _____

Lotto Game

Matching

Instructor: Reproduce two copies of the lotto game for each child. Have the child color the picture, then cut apart one set of them. The children can then match the pictures.

Turkey-O

Instructor: Reproduce two copies of the lotto game for each child .One will be cut apart to make a "deck" of pictures. The child needs 12 markers (blocks, counters, chips, small squares of construction paper).

The instructor says, "Listen carefully. I will pick a card and name the picture. You find the picture and put a marker on it."

Other Suggestions/Activities

- The instructor can pick a card and give a clue, description, or riddle about the picture. The child places a marker on the picture he thinks goes with the clues.

- In a group situation, the children can take turns picking a card and either naming it or giving a clue to the other children.

- Place the lotto game and deck of cards in a learning center. Color, paste on cardboard and laminate.

Lotto Game

Thanksgiving - Worksheet 15

TURKEY-O

Name _____ Date _____

Turkey Tails

Thanksgiving - Worksheet 16

Yes/No Questions

Instructor: "Listen carefully. I will tell you something. If I am right, answer yes. If I am wrong, answer no."
When the child's response is correct, a feather on the turkey's tail can be colored.

1. Pilgrims wore hats. (yes)
2. The Pilgrims came to America on an airplane. (no)
3. The Indians and Pilgrims made friends. (yes)
4. The Pilgrims bought their crops. (no)
5. Corn was one of their crops. (yes)
6. Apples are vegetables. (no)
7. Pie can be eaten for dessert. (yes)
8. A turkey has fur. (no)
9. A tree can grow tall. (yes)
10. A leaf is part of a car. (no)
11. Acorns grow on apple trees. (no)
12. Squirrels like to eat acorns. (yes)

Sentence Completion

Instructor: "Listen carefully. I will say part of a sentence. When I stop, you say a word to finish the sentence." When the child's response is correct, a feather on the turkey's tail can be colored.

1. A turkey is a _____. (bird)
2. A ship travels on _____. (water)
3. An apple is a _____. (fruit)
4. An acorn comes from an oak _____. (tree)
5. A squirrel has a bushy _____. (tail)
6. The Pilgrims came to America on a _____. (ship)
7. Corn is a _____. (vegetable)
8. You wear a hat on your_____. (head)
9. A tree is a _____. (plant)
10. A pie is baked in the _____. (oven)
11. Indians helped the Pilgrims plant _____. (crops)
12. A leaf comes from a _____. (tree)

Turkey Tails

Thanksgiving - Worksheet 16

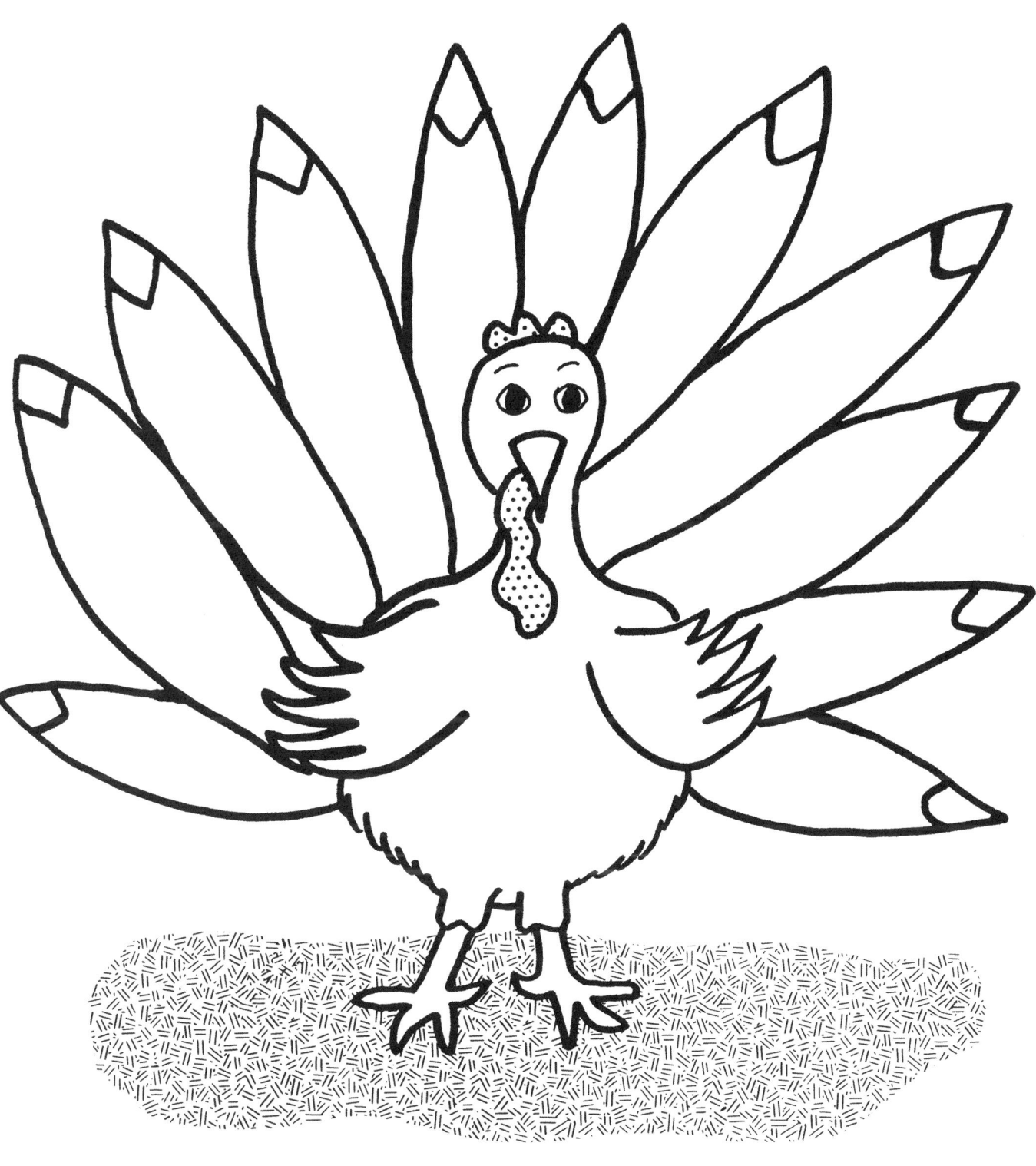

Name _____ Date _____

Tree Time

<u>**Instructor**</u>: Discuss how the leaves on trees change colors and then begin to fall off the trees. Have child observe trees outside. Which trees are losing their leaves?

<u>Sequence Activity</u>

Have child color and cut out each picture. The child can put the pictures in order and paste on construction paper.

<u>Listen and Say</u>

<u>**Instructor**</u>: This activity allows a child to listen to a question and then immediately respond. Read the statement, then ask the child the question.

1. A tree is a plant.
   What is a tree?

2. A tree has a trunk.
   What does a tree have?

3. The leaves on trees change colors.
   What do the leaves do?

4. Trees lose their leaves in the fall.
   When do trees lose their leaves?

5. A tree can grow tall.
   How can a tree grow?

<u>Other Suggestions/Activities</u>

- Have the child collect leaves from trees outside. Have child paste leaves on construction paper for a collage. Use tracing paper and have child make a crayon tracing of the leaf.

- Have the child observe a tree and draw a picture.

Tree Time

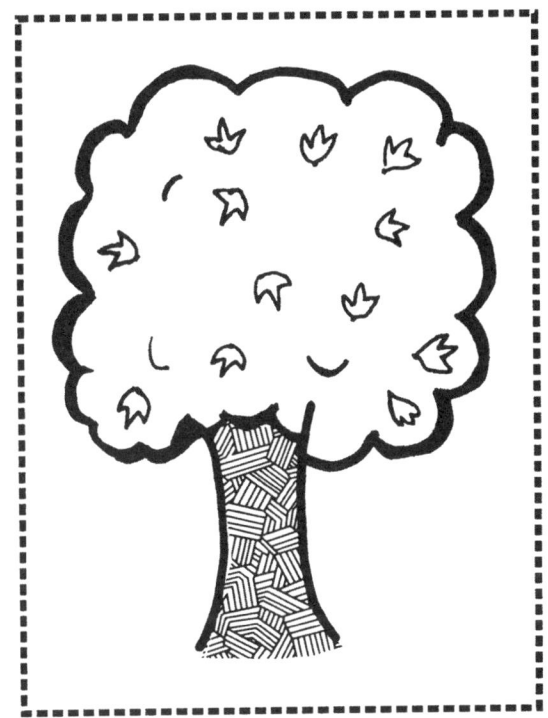

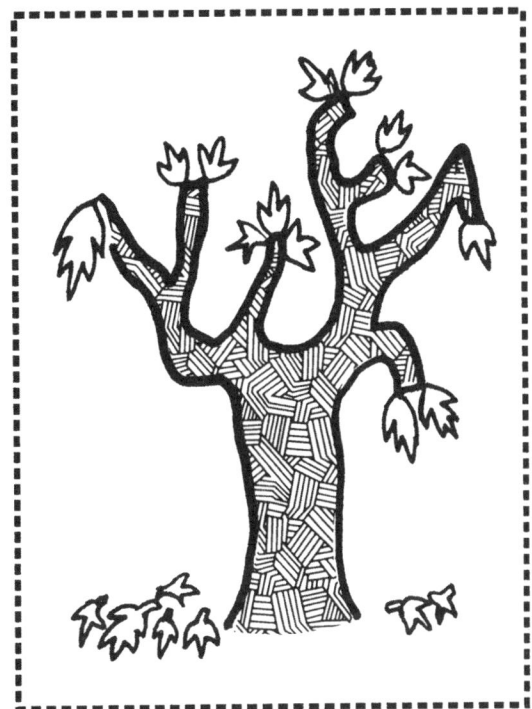

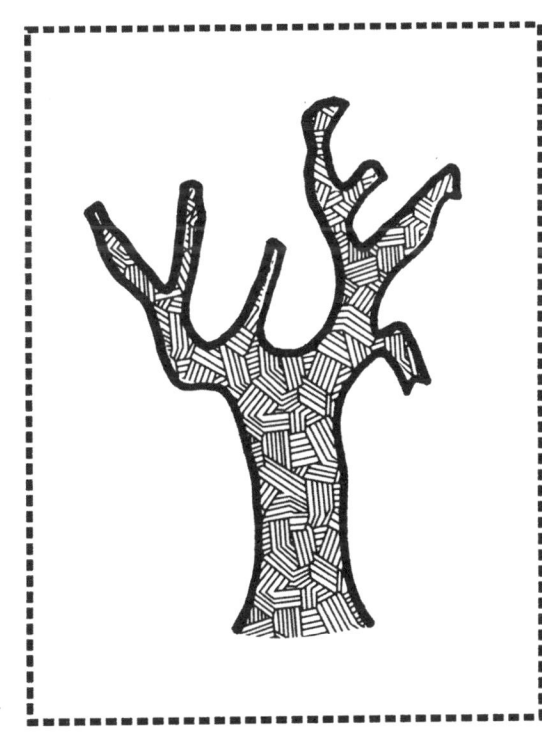

Visual Discrimination - Motor Activity

Instructor: Have the child examine each picture individually. Have child tell you what is missing. If the child needs help getting started, try the following:

Ex: "A ship needs sails to move through the water. Look carefully at the ship. Is anything missing?"

After the child tells you what is missing from each picture, have him draw the missing items on the pictures.

Auditory Discrimination

Instructor: "Listen carefully and do as I say."

Draw some tail feathers on the turkey.

Draw a hat on the Pilgrim.

Draw some sails for the ship.

Draw some eyes on the Indian.

Draw a tail on the squirrel.

Other Suggestions/Activities

- Use for the development of basic concept words. Ex: Draw a line <u>under</u> the Pilgrim, draw a square <u>over</u> the squirrel.

- Use for "I am Thinking" game. The instructor says, "I am thinking of an animal. It is a bird. It has feathers. What is it?"

Following Directions

Thanksgiving - Worksheet 18

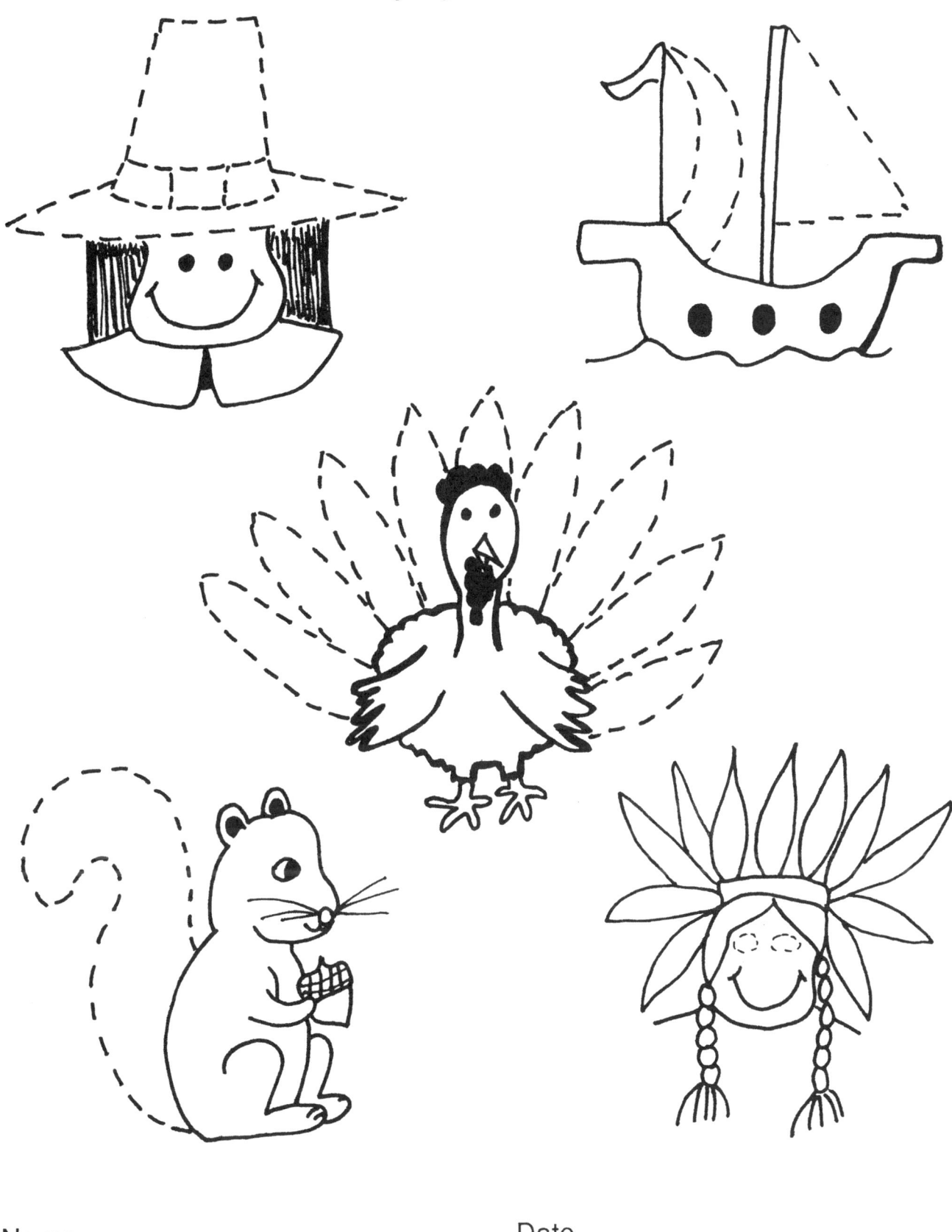

Name _____   Date _____

41

Five Little Squirrels

Instructor: Have the child color and cut out the squirrels. Read the "Five Little Squirrels" poem below. As you say each verse, have the child paste a squirrel on the worksheet.

Five Little Squirrels

One little squirrel in the old oak tree,
Gathering acorns - as busy as can be.

Two little squirrels in the old oak tree,
Helping each other, can't you see?

Three little squirrels in the old oak tree,
Working, working, just like you and me.

Four little squirrels in the old oak tree,
Much too busy to even stop for tea.

Five little squirrels in the old oak tree,
Finished for the day at half past three.

Position Words

Instructor: Have the child color and cut out the squirrels. Tell the child, "Listen carefully and do what I say."

"Paste (put) a squirrel in the tree."

"Put a squirrel under the tree."

"Put a squirrel by the tree."

"Put a squirrel on the tree trunk."

"Put a squirrel on the ground."

Other Suggestions/Activities

- Number the squirrels 1 - 5. Have the child practice counting.

- Use the poem with the squirrel stick puppet (page 49). Have the child learn this poem and recite it. The five squirrels on page 43 may also be used as stick puppets.

Five Little Squirrels

Thanksgiving - Worksheet 19

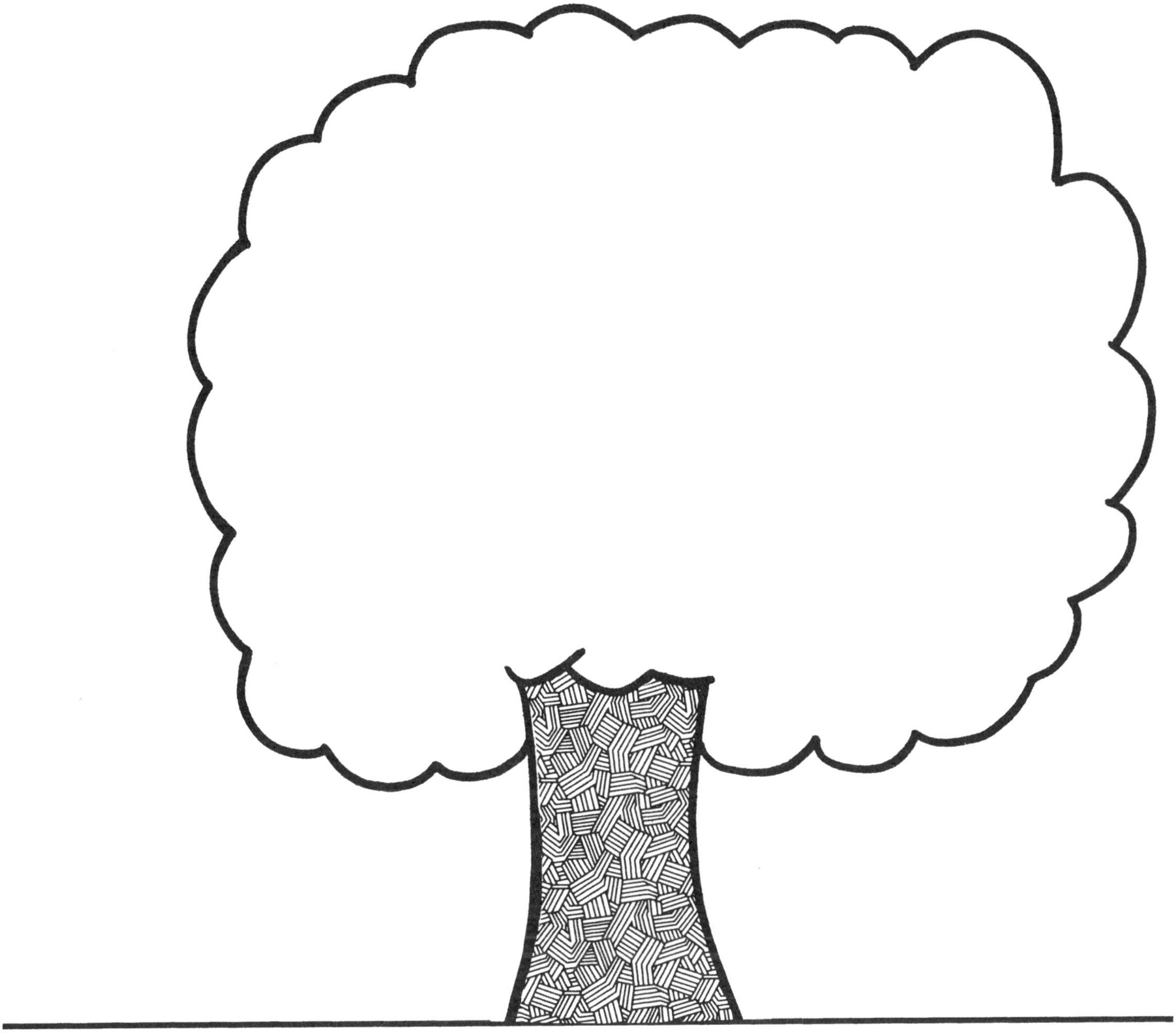

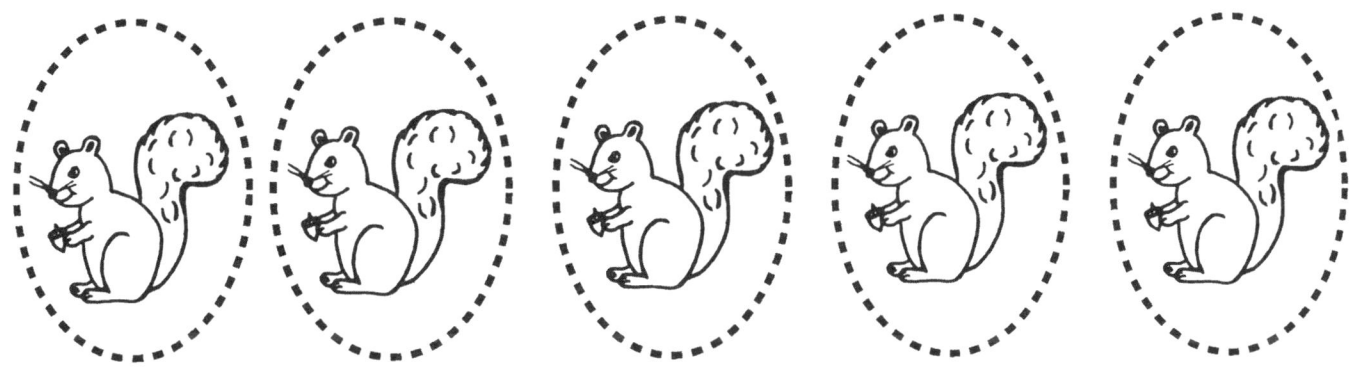

Thanksgiving Story

Instructor: Read "Ann's Thanksgiving Visit" to child. If possible, use props to assist in attending skills. (Dress up like a Pilgrim or Indian, place a bowl of fruits and vegetables near by, or construct a Pilgrim collar, (page 51).

Storytime

Reproduce stick puppets (page 49). Have the child color, cut out, and paste on a tongue depressor or popsicle stick. Use while telling the story or have the child hold up a stick puppet when they hear the name of their character in the story. Use the stick puppets and have the child retell a part of the story.

Other Suggestions/Activities

- Read one paragraph at a time and ask "WH" questions.

> Ex: Paragraph 1
> What day was it?
> Why did Ann get up early?
> Why didn't Ann have to go to school?

- Have the child draw a picture about the story and tell about the picture.

Ann's Thanksgiving Visit

Characters: Ann, Mother, Muffin (cat)

Ann gets up early this cool Thursday morning. It's a special fall holiday. "Why are you up so early? There is no school today," says Mother. "Today is special. You have a day off from work and we can be together," says Ann. "Our time together is very special for me too," says Mother.

"Let's talk while you eat your cereal. Today is going to be special because we are going to see Grandmother and Grandfather. This is the fourth Thursday in November, " Mother says. "It's Thanksgiving!" says Ann. "I bet Granny has been cooking for days because all the relatives are coming for Thanksgiving dinner." "Let's get ready to go to Granny's," says Mother.

Ann is getting ready for the big day. She is thinking about what to wear. She is talking to Muffin, her cat. "First, I put on my new blue dress with long sleeves. Second, I put on my shoes. Now, I put on my coat. I put my hat on last. I want to dress in warm clothes because we have cool weather in November," says Ann. "Meow," says Muffin.

Ann says goodbye to Muffin as she leaves for Granny's house. "Here is some special cat food for you. Thanksgiving is special for everyone. Be sweet and take a nap while we are gone," says Ann. "Meow, meow," says Muffin.

Ann and Mother are riding in the car. "Let's talk about the first Thanksgiving," says Mother. "The Pilgrims came to America from another country. They rode on a ship across the sea. The Mayflower was the name of the ship. When they got to America they built houses and planted crops. The Pilgrims were happy. They would have food to eat all winter. They wanted to celebrate with a big party. They invited some of their Indian friends. They ate many different foods. They ate meat, vegetables, and fruits. They ate beans, corn, pumpkin pie and apples. They ate outside."

"The first Thanksgiving was like a great big picnic. We celebrate every year with our family and friends. You and I go to Granny's every year

45

to see Grandpa and your aunts, uncles, and cousins," says Mother. "Many people travel a very long way to see their families at Thanksgiving. Some people drive many miles in a car. Others fly on an airplane or ride a train or bus. Thanksgiving is a very special holiday," says Mother.

Ann says, "At school we made special hats. Some were like Pilgrims. Some were like Indians. We made a special Thanksgiving dinner. The teacher brought a special slow cooking pot to school. All the children took cans of food. I took corn. We made soup by putting all the food in the pot. It cooked all morning. We ate our Thanksgiving meal. We had paper bowls. The teacher said the Pilgrims had wooden bowls. We wore our Pilgrim and Indian hats. It was fun."

Ann and Mother finally get to Granny's house. There are lots of people. Everyone is smiling and happy to see Ann. Ann hugs her Granny and Grandpa first. "Wow! Smell the food. Look at all the good things to eat. We have beans, corn and carrots. I like to eat apples and pumpkin pie. What a feast," says Ann.

"My Mom made us special hats to wear today," says cousin Dan. "She made a Pilgrim hat and Indian hat." "We need one more," says Ann. "Why?" says Dan. "We need a hat for the turkey," Ann says. "He forgot his feathers!"

Thanksgiving Story - Stick Puppets
Thanksgiving - Worksheet 20

Instructions: Have child color then cut out each character. Paste each character to the end of a tongue depressor or popsicle stick.

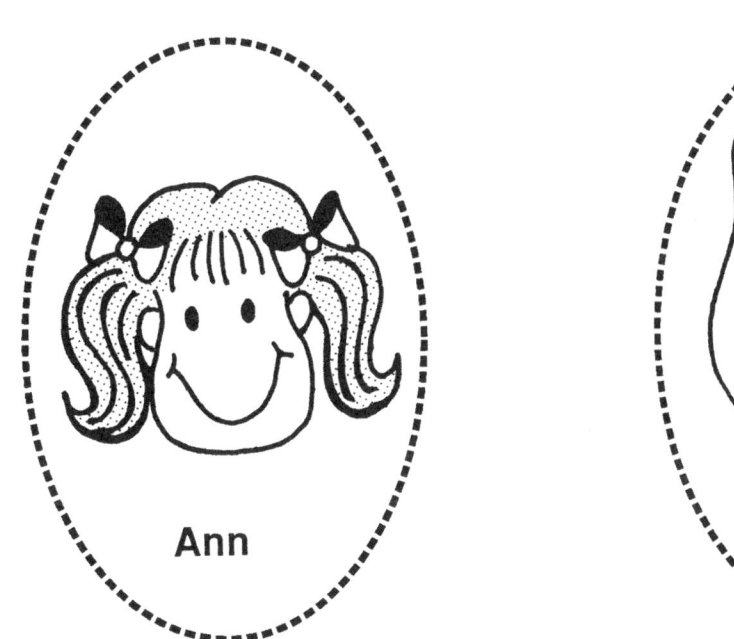

Ann

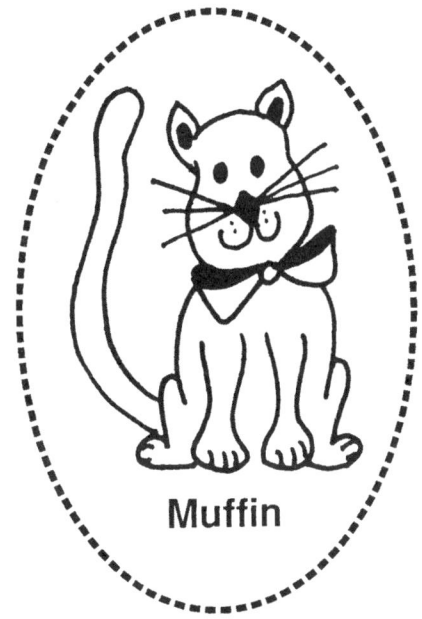

Muffin

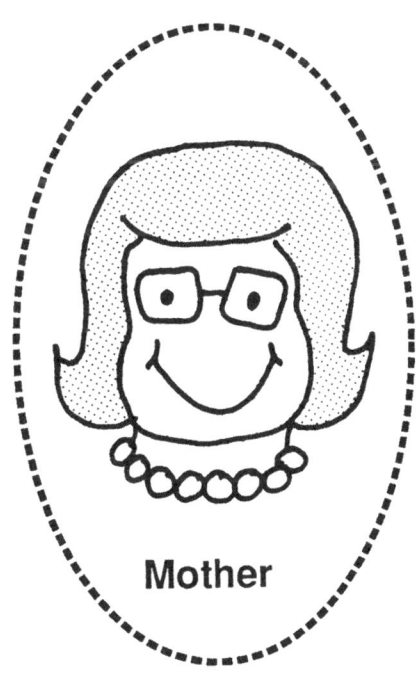

Mother

Rhyming Time

Instructor: Reproduce stick puppets (page 49). Have the child color and cut out. Paste each character to the end of a tongue depressor or popicle stick. Read a poem. Have the child hold up a stick puppet when they hear the name of their character.

Poem Time

Pilgrims

The Pilgrims' ship,
Sailed on the sea.
They made the trip,
For you and me.

The Indian

The Indian walked,
Across the ground.
The Indian walked
Without a sound.

The Squirrel

The squirrel's tail,
Helps him sail,
Through the trees,
Like a breeze.

Thanksgiving

Thanksgiving is coming,
The turkeys are running.
Run little turkey - - as fast as you can,
You don't want - - to end up in the pan.

Squirrel

The little squirrel ran up the tree,
He ran so fast he was hard to see.
He grabbed an acorn - - big and brown,
He looked around, then ran back down.

Other Suggestions/Activities

- Sentence completion. Read a poem and leave of the last word in the line.
 Have the child complete the line by saying the word.

- Have the child learn one poem and recite it using a stick puppet.

- Rewrite a poem on large chart paper. Have the child draw a picture to go with
 the poem. Place on bulletin board.

Rhyming Time - Stick Puppets

Thanksgiving - Worksheet 21

Instructions: Have child color then cut out each character. Paste each character to the end of a tongue depressor or popsicle stick.

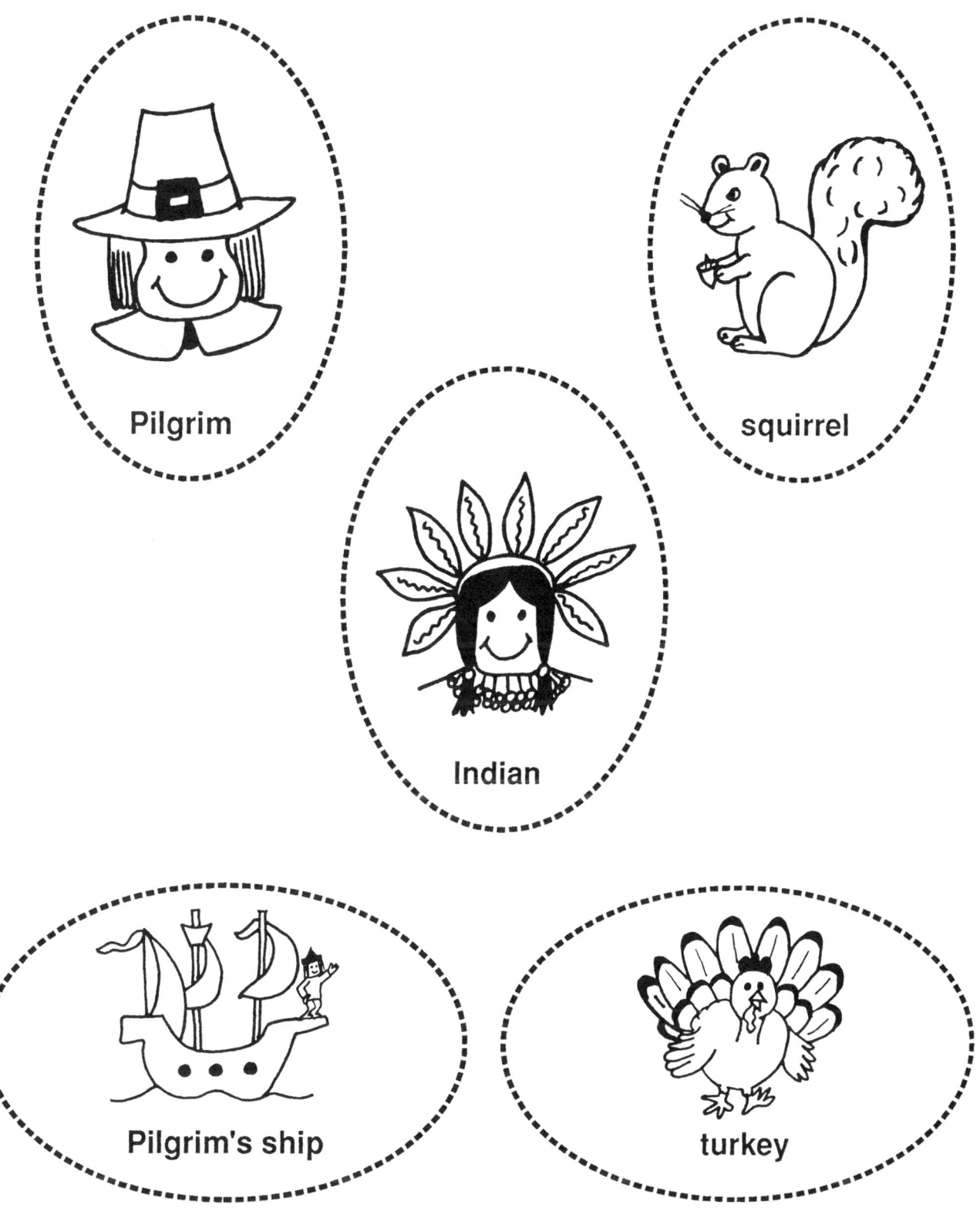

Pilgrim

squirrel

Indian

Pilgrim's ship

turkey

Time for a Play

Instructor: Use the patterns on page 51. Have the child choose and make either the Pilgrim collar or the Indian vest. Have the child act out or tell about his character.

Short Play

Instructor: Have the children make three Indian vests and two Pilgrim collars. Have children perform play.

Indian 1 -   Hello! Where are you from?

Pilgrim 1 -   We are from another country.

Indian 2 -   We will be your friends.

Pilgrim 2 -   Can you show us how to plant our crops?

Indian 3 -   Yes. We will help you hunt and fish, too.

(All shake hands)

Other Suggestions/Activities

- Have the child say a poem or riddle about his character.

- Circle Story: Have children sit in a circle. Tell the first child a story beginning and have the child continue the story. When the first child has said a sentence or two, have the next child continue the story. The story continues around the circle with each child adding to it.

Story beginnings: Once there was a Pilgrim and.....................................

A turkey was walking down a road and........................

An Indian was walking through the forest and.............

Time for a Play

Indian Vest

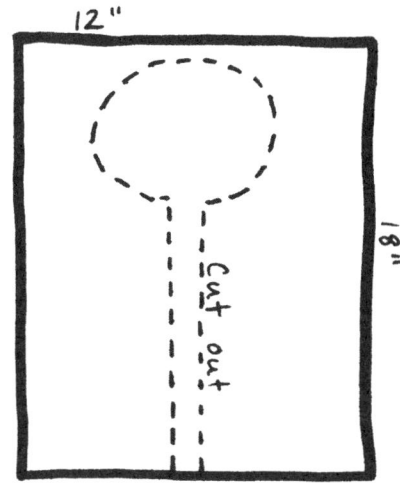 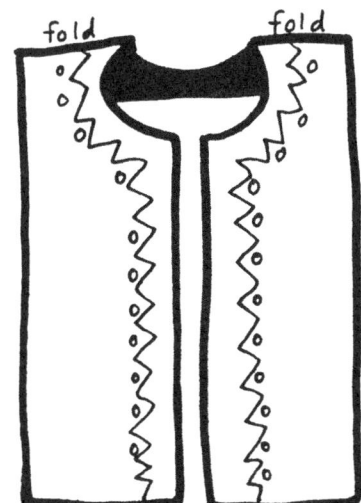

Directions: Use a 12" x 18" piece of brown construction paper. Draw a 6" circle one inch from top end. This is the neck opening. Cut a one inch strip out of the front from the bottom to the neck circle. This is the front opening. Cut out the neck circle. Fit vest around child's neck. Fold slightly to make it hang over shoulders. Have the child decorate the vest.

Pilgrim Collar

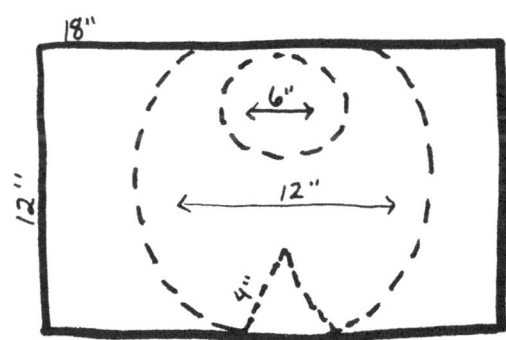 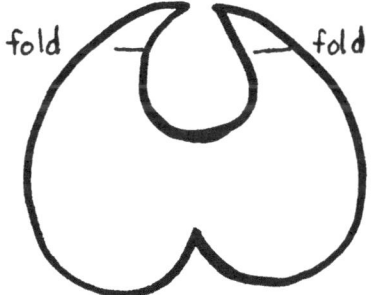

Directions: Use a 12" x 18" piece of white construction paper. Draw a 12" circle. Draw a 6" circle close to edge for the neck opening. Draw a 4" triangle for front of collar. Cut out collar, neck opening, and front triangle. Fold slightly to make collar fit over shoulders. Fasten in back with tape.

Let's Talk About Christmas

Introduction to Christmas

Instructor: Tell the child about Christmas.

Ex: Christmas is a holiday that we celebrate in December. It is on December 25th. People celebrate this as the birthdate of Jesus. During the Christmas season people decorate their homes and put up a Christmas tree. They put decorations on the tree. They may put a pretty wreath on the door or lights in the windows. They give presents to their friends and family. They make food to give to others. Christmas comes in winter. The weather can be very cold and snowy. Children can have fun playing outside with sleds or making a snowman.

Core Vocabulary

Use the picture cards (pages 54 and 55) to introduce the Christmas core vocabulary. Have the child color the pictures. The pictures may be cut out and mounted on light cardboard. Describe each picture. Tell about the size, color, or particular attributes of each object.

Match-up Activity

Reproduce two of each picture to make a set. Have the child find the matching pictures after you have scrambled them.

Memory Game

Place two to four cards on the table. Have the child look at the cards for a few seconds. Cover or turn them over. Have the child name the pictures from memory.

Other Suggestions/Activities

- Reproduce the picture cards. Use with the gameboard on page 77. Have the child name or describe picture before moving.

- Reproduce two of each picture. Use to play concentration game.

- Use the cards to reinforce preposition concepts. Ex: Instructor says, "Put the star under your chair." "Put the snowman beside your chair."

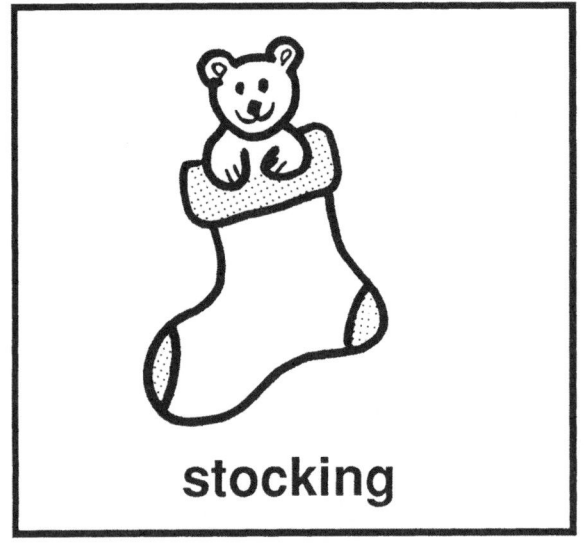

stocking

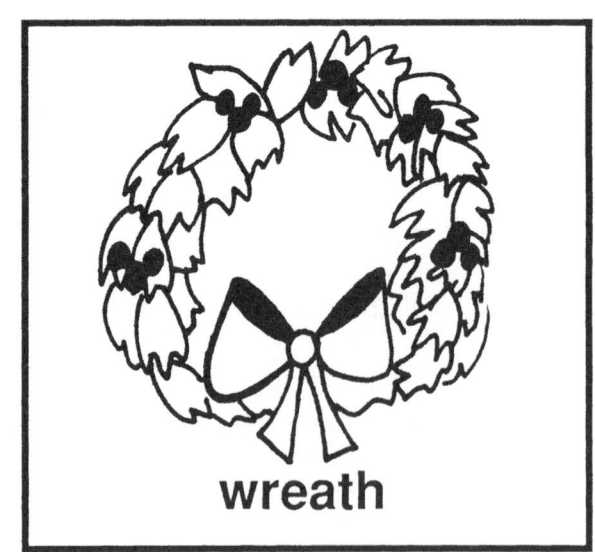

wreath

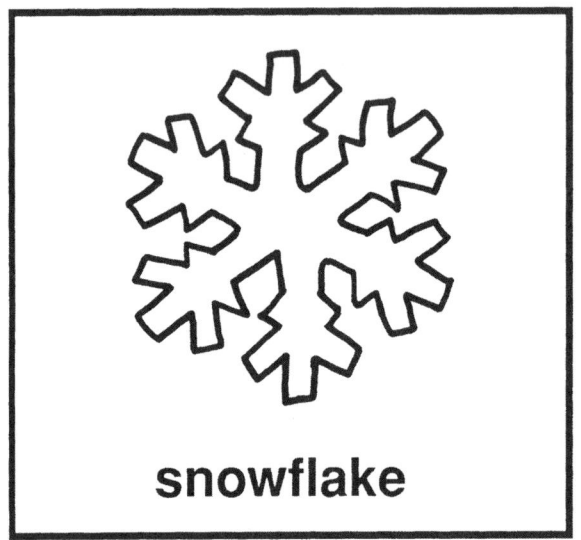

snowflake

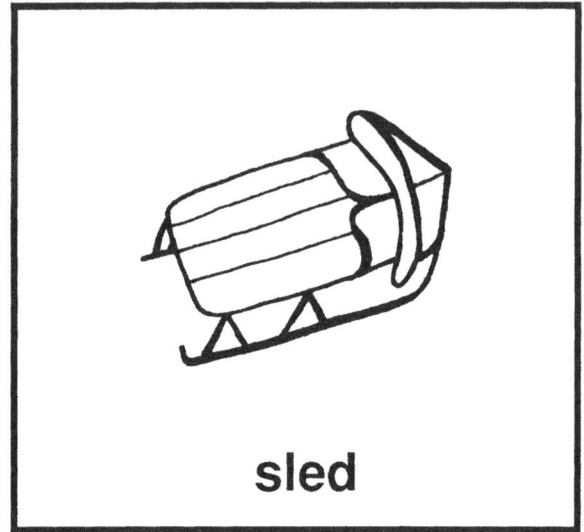

sled

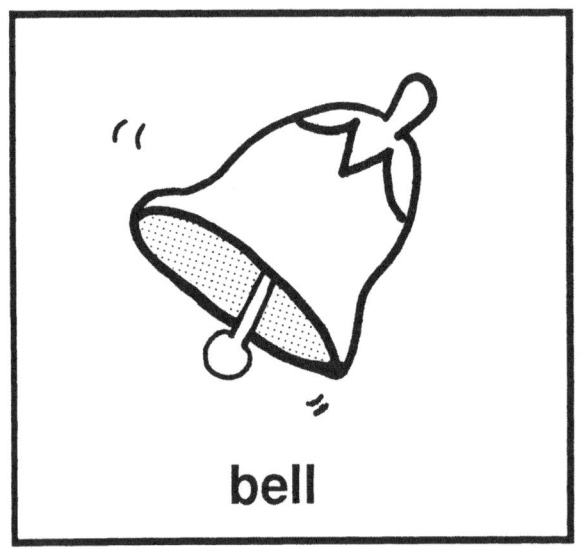

bell

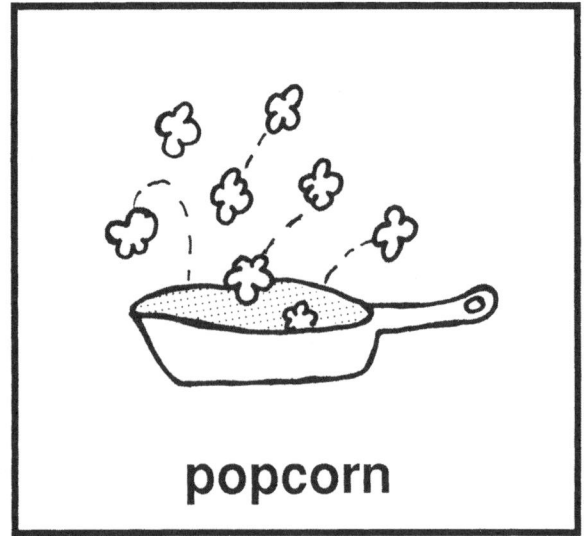

popcorn

54

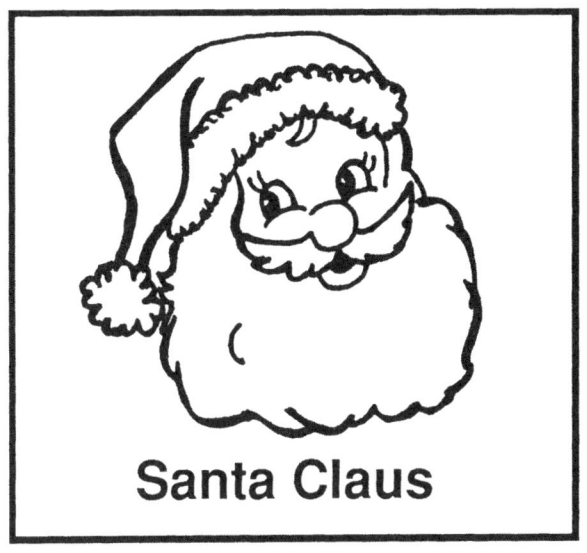

Santa Claus

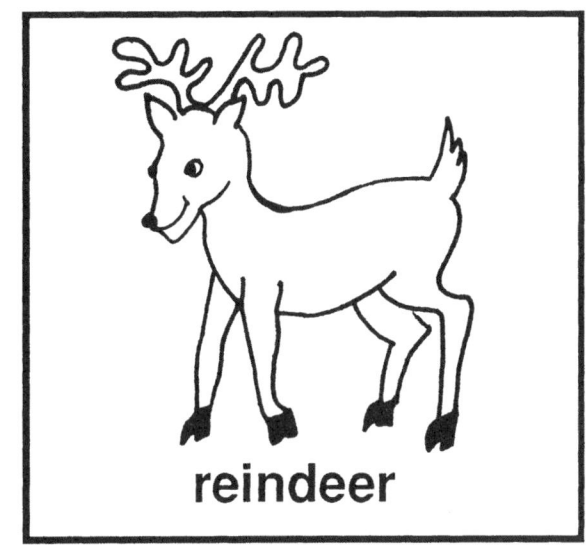

reindeer

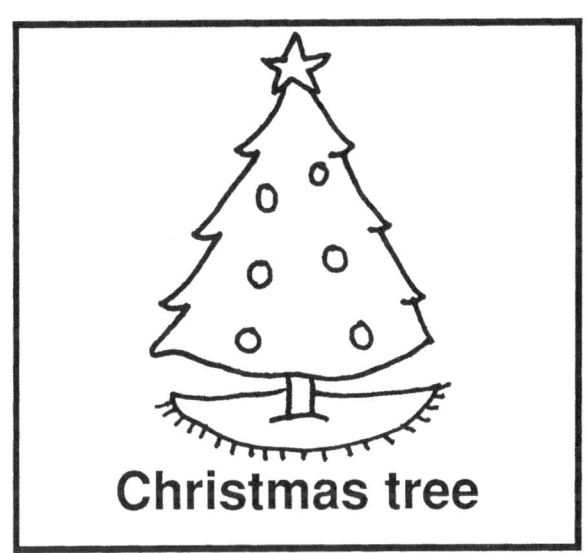

Christmas tree

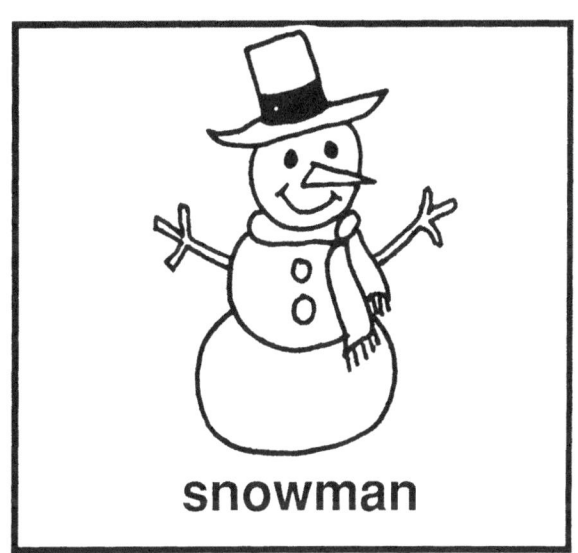

snowman

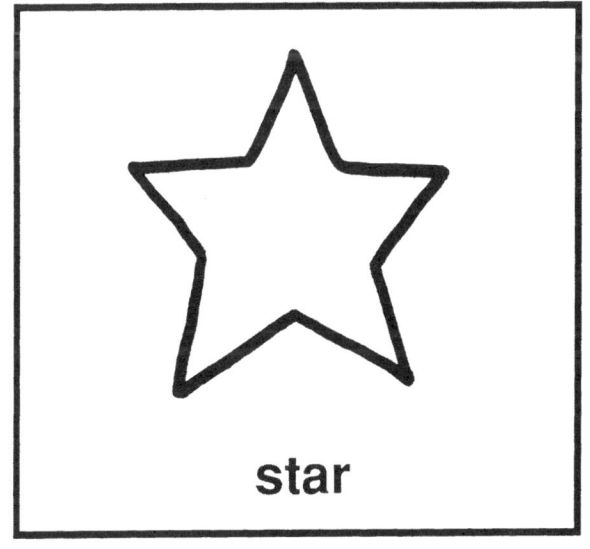

star

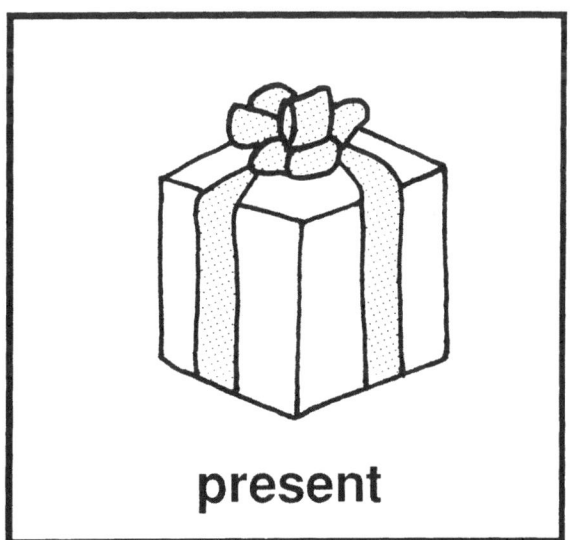

present

55

Riddle Time

Instructor: Read each riddle below. Have the child choose which picture is being described. When the child chooses correctly, the picture can be colored.

1. He is a person
   He has a white beard.
   He wears a red suit.
   He drives a sleigh.
   He says, "Ho, Ho, Ho."
   Who is he? (Santa Claus)

2. It is an animal.
   It has antlers.
   It has four legs.
   It lives in cold places.
   What is it? (reindeer)

3. It grows outside.
   It is a plant.
   It is always green.
   It is tall.
   You put decorations on it.
   What is it? (Christmas tree)

4. It has 5 points.
   It is shiny.
   You can put it on your
     Christmas tree.
   What is it? (star)

5. It is wrapped in pretty paper.
   It has a bow on it.
   You give it to someone else.
   It has a surprise inside.
   What is it? (present)

6. It is made of cloth.
   It is shaped like a sock.
   You can hang it up.
   Santa puts surprises in it.
   What is it? (stocking)

7. You can hang it on your tree.
   It is made of metal.
   It makes a sound.
   It jingles or goes ding-dong.
   What is it? (bell)

8. You can hang it on your door
     or in your house.
   It is made from green plants.
   It has a bow on it.
   It is shaped like a circle.
   What is it? (wreath)

9. It is something to eat.
   It is white and little.
   It comes from corn.
   When you heat it, it pops open.
   It tastes salty.
   What is it? (popcorn)

10. You ride on this.
    It goes fast.
    It has runners.
    You use it when it snows.
    What is it? (sled)

11. It is made of frozen rain.
    It falls from clouds.
    It is white.
    It is light as a feather.
    What is it? (snow)

12. It is made of snow.
    It looks like a person.
    It has a head and body.
    It stays outside.
    Children make this in winter.
    What is it? (snowman)

Other Suggestions/Activities

- Use the Christmas scene to talk about Christmas.

- Have the child color the Christmas scene and then tell a story about it.

- Have the child color and name all the objects in the scene.

Riddle Time

Christmas-Worksheet 24

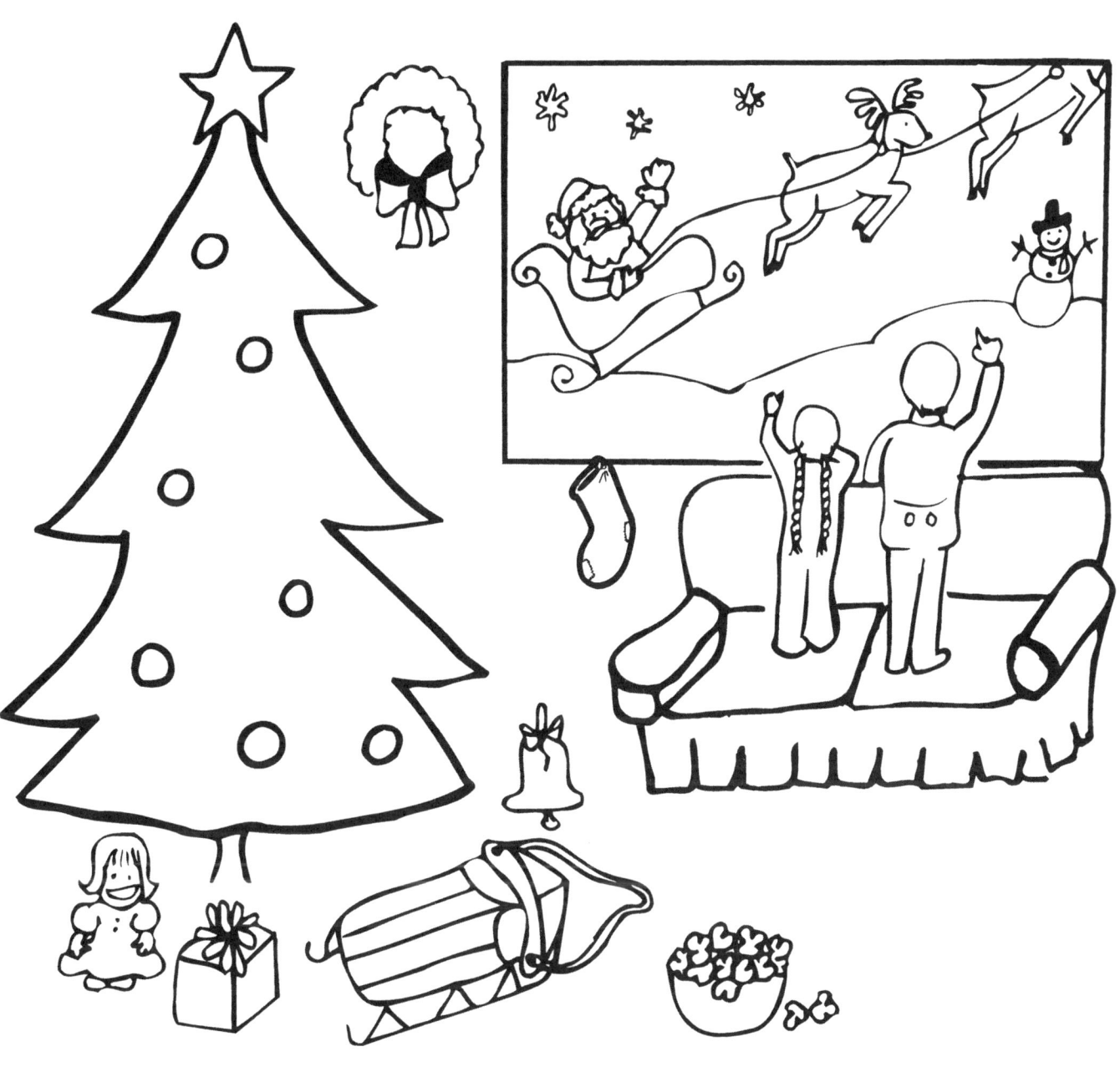

Name _____ Date _____

Spin a Word

Christmas - Worksheet 25

Instructor: Have the child color and cut out spinner. Paste on heavy cardboard. Use a brad to connect the spinner.

Listen and Say

Instructor: "After you spin, I will ask you a question about your word."

(snowflake)	1. How does a snowflake feel?
(Santa Claus)	2. What does Santa Claus say?
(reindeer)	3. What do reindeers pull?
(Christmas tree)	4. What do we put on a Christmas tree?
(snowman)	5. What is a snowman made from?
(present)	6. What do you do with a present?
(star)	7. How does a star look?
(stocking)	8. What does Santa put in a stocking?
(bell)	9. What sound does a bell make?
(wreath)	10. Where can you hang a wreath?
(popcorn)	11. How does popcorn taste?
(sled)	12. Where do you ride a sled?

Other Suggestions/Activities

- The child spins and tells about the picture.

> Ex: It is an animal.
> It has 4 legs.
> It pulls Santa's sleigh.
> It has antlers.

- The child spins and gives a description of his picture not giving the name. The other children guess what picture is being described.

- The child spins and uses the word in a short sentence.

Spin a Word

Christmas - Worksheet 25

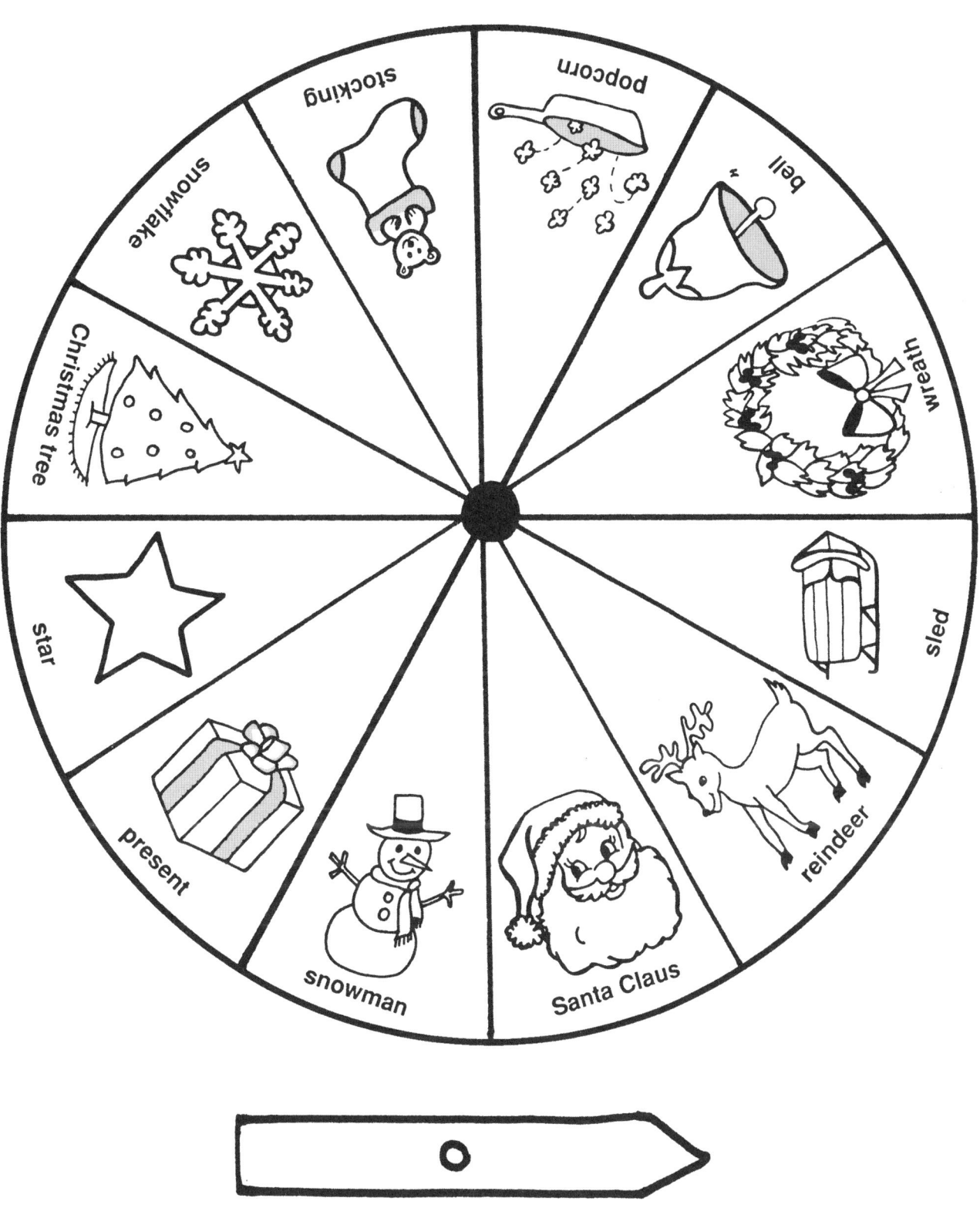

Mr. Snowman

Instructor: Discuss the weather and activities associated with snow. Talk about making a snowman and what happens first, next, and last.

Sequence Activity

Have child color and cut out each picture. The child can put them in order and paste on construction paper.

Listen and Say

Instructor: This activity allows a child to listen to a question and then immediately respond. Read the statement, then ask the child the question.

1. A snowman is made from snowballs.
   What is a snowman made from?

2. We make snowmen in winter.
   When do we make snowmen?

3. We need three snowballs to make a snowman.
   How many snowballs do we need?

4. We can put a hat on a snowman.
   What can we put on a snowman?

5. The sun will make the snowman melt.
   What will make the snowman melt?

Other Suggestions/Activities

- Have the child dictate a short story about the sequence pictures. Place story and sequence pictures on bulletin board.

Mr. Snowman

Christmas - Worksheet 26

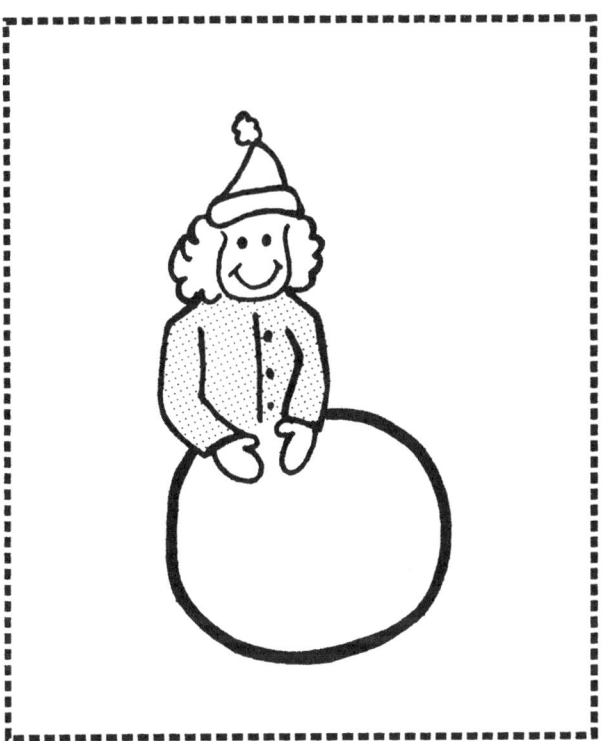 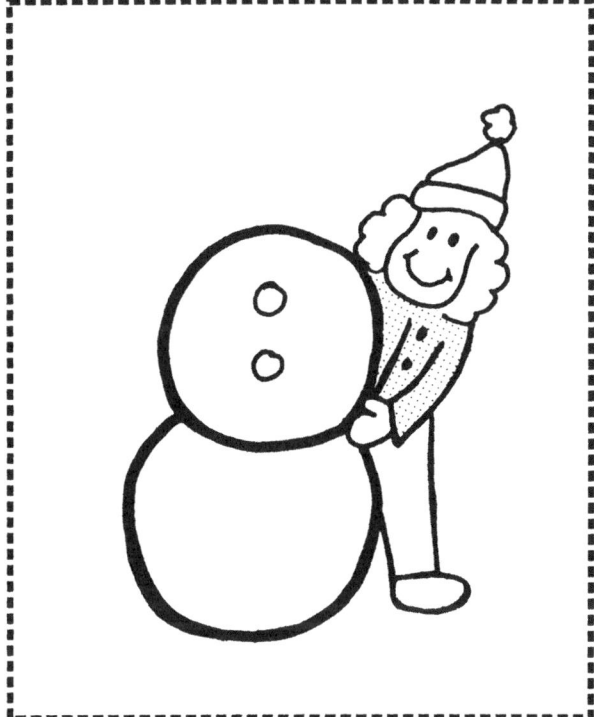

 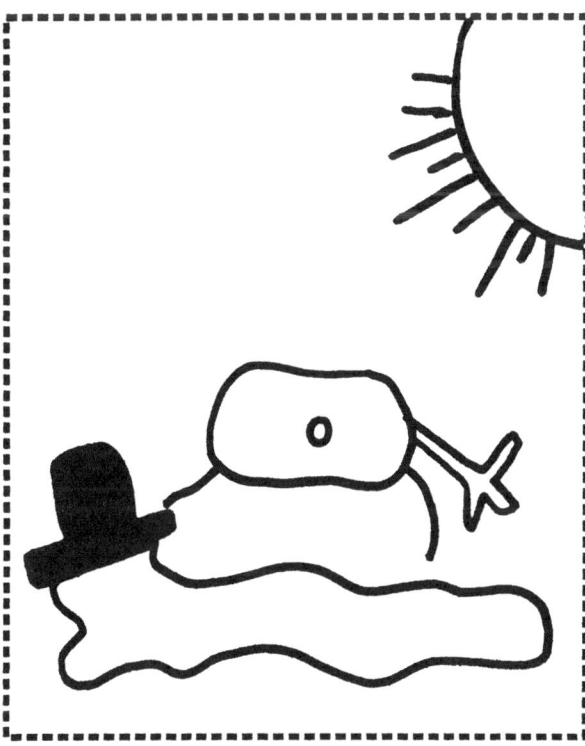

Following Directions

<u>Instructor</u>: Have the child examine each picture individually. Have the child tell you what is missing. If the child needs help getting started, try the following:

Ex: "Santa usually wears something on his head. It is red. Look carefully at this Santa. Is anything missing?"

After the child tells you what is missing from each picture have him draw the missing items on the pictures.

Auditory Discrimination

<u>Instructor</u>: "Listen carefully and do as I say."

"Draw some antlers on the reindeer."

"Draw a cap for Santa."

"Draw some eyes for the snowman."

"Draw some decorations on the tree."

"Draw a bow on the present."

Other Suggestions/Activities

- Use for the development of basic concept words.

Ex: Draw a line <u>under</u> the reindeer. Draw a circle <u>over</u> the snowman.

- Use for "I am Thinking Game." The instructor says, "I am thinking of an animal. It is brown. It has antlers. It has four legs. It pulls Santa's sleigh. What is it?"

Following Directions

Christmas - Worksheet 27

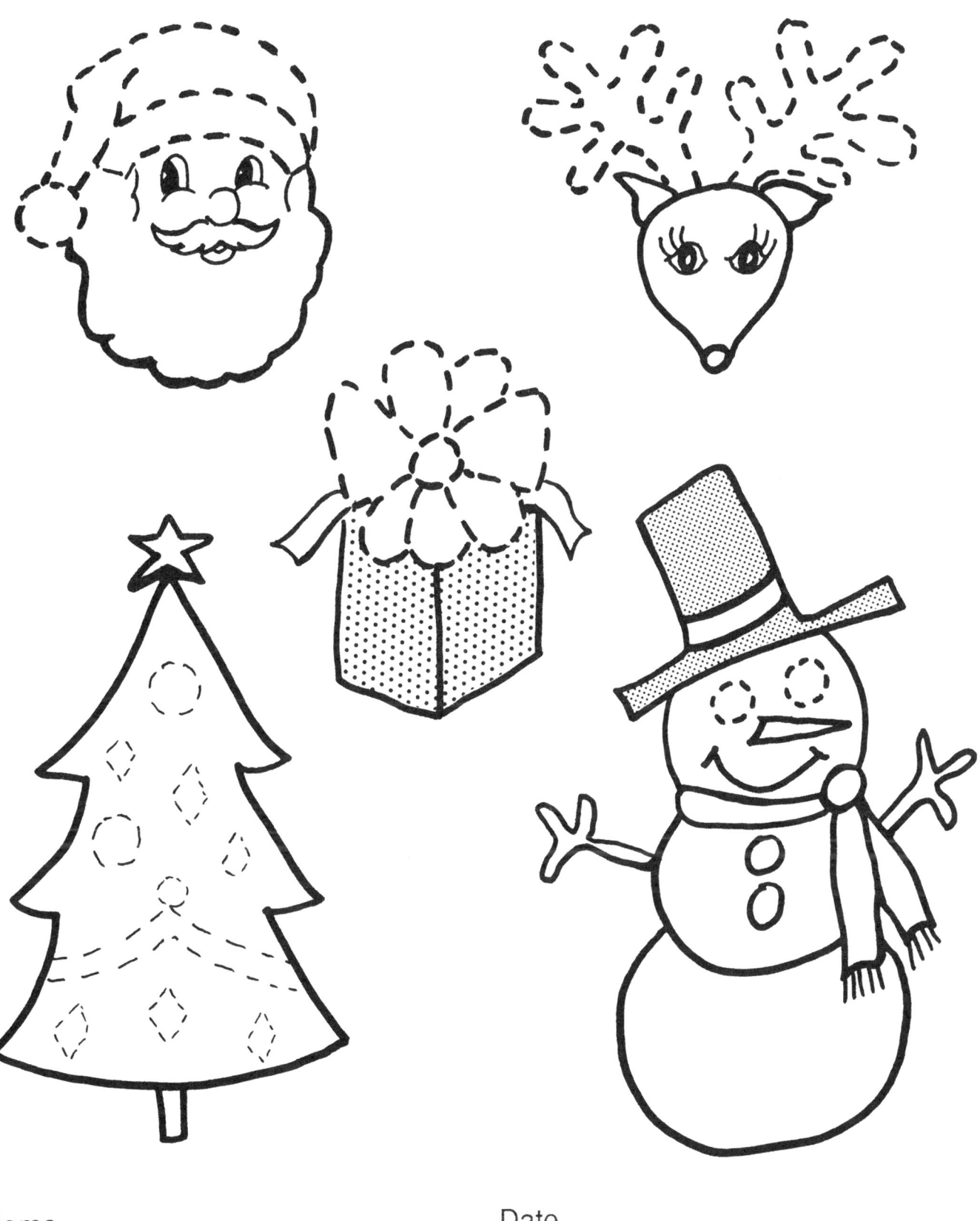

Name _____   Date _____

Decorate the Tree

Christmas - Worksheet 28

Yes/No Questions

Instructor: "Listen carefully. I will tell you something. If I am right, answer YES.
If I am wrong, answer NO." (When the child's response is correct,
a decoration can be colored on the tree.)

1. Santa rides in a sleigh. (yes)

2. Reindeers have 4 legs. (yes)

3. Christmas trees are black. (no)

4. A star is round. (no)

5. We give presents to others. (yes)

6. You put your stocking under the bed. (no)

7. Bells go beep, beep. (no)

8. A wreath is shaped like a circle. (yes)

9. Popcorn makes a sound when it pops. (yes)

10. A snowflake is hot. (no)

11. We ride a sled down a hill. (yes)

12. A snowman is made of snowballs. (yes)

Sentence Completion

Instructor: "Listen carefully. I will say a part of a sentence. When I stop, you say
a word to finish the sentence. (When the child's response is correct,
a decoration can be colored on the tree.)

1. Santa comes on _____. (Christmas)

2. Reindeers have four _____. (legs)

3. Evergreens are always _____. (green)

4. We can put a star at the top of our _____. (tree)

5. Ribbon and wrapping paper cover a _____. (present)

6. A stocking can be filled with _____. (toys, surprises)

7. A bell goes _____. (jingle, jingle, ding/dong)

8. A wreath is shaped like a _____. (circle)

9. We can string popcorn with a needle and _____. (thread)

10. Snowflakes fall from _____. (clouds)

11. We can ride a sled in the _____. (snow)

12. A snowman is made of _____. (snowballs, snow)

Other Suggestions/Activities

- Duplicate the tree pattern on green construction paper. Provide small pieces of lace, ribbon, gummed stickers or stars. Have the child decorate the tree.

- Duplicate two tree patterns on green construction paper. Have the child decorate all sides of the patterns using crayons and then cut out each tree. Place the two trees together and staple lengthwise down the middle in four or five places. Fold out to make a three dimensional tree.

Decorate the Tree

Christmas - Worksheet 28

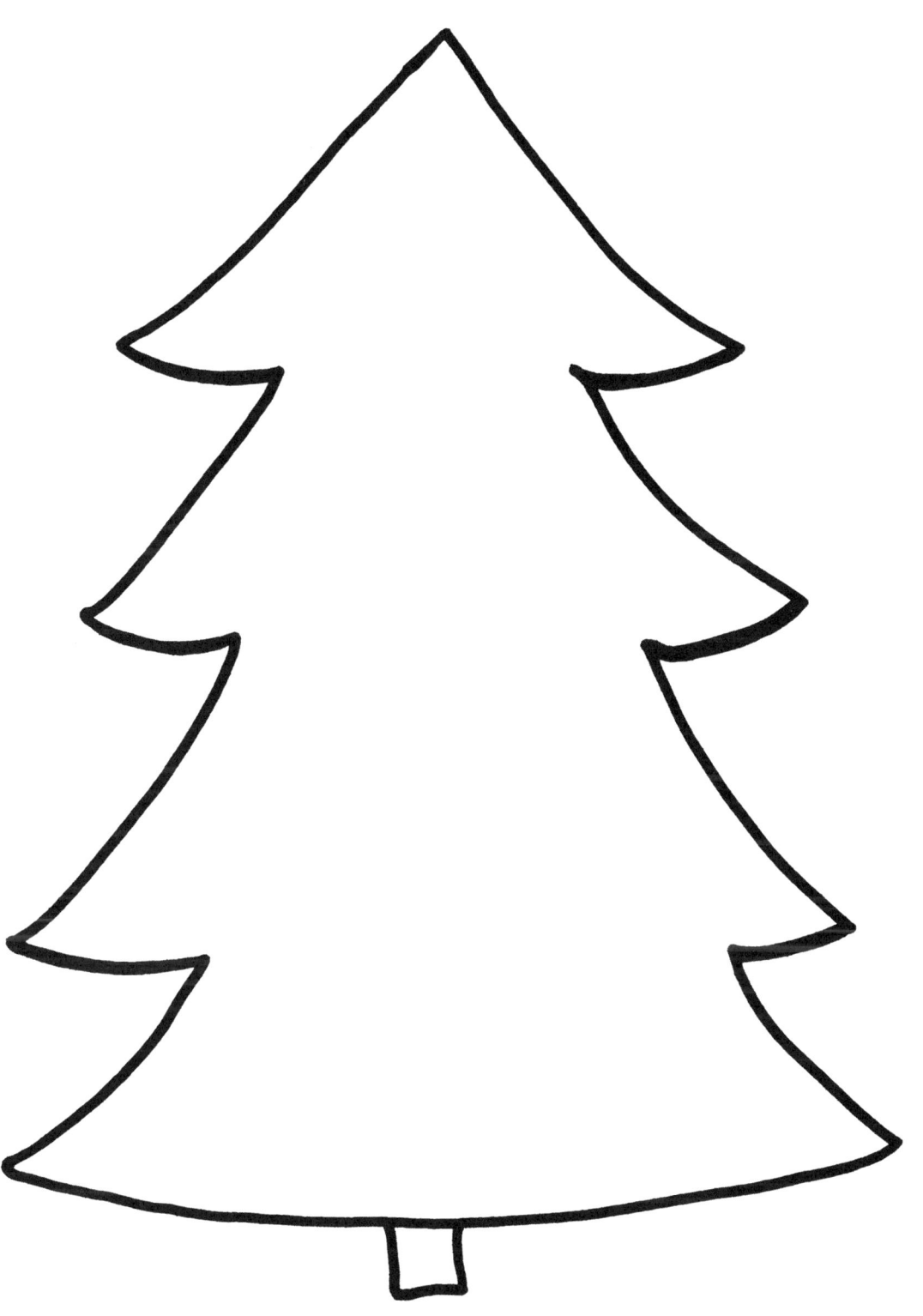

Name _____   Date _____

65

Using Your Senses
Christmas - Worksheet 29

Instructor: Discuss each picture with the child. Talk about what it looks, sounds, smells, feels, or tastes like. If possible, have samples or objects to listen to, smell, feel, or taste. (i.e. popcorn, pine needles or cedar, piece of ice, small bell, 2 blocks to hit together for reindeer on roof, cellophane for crackling fire.)

Using Your Senses

Instructor: "I will tell you about a picture. Close your eyes and listen. When I finish, open your eyes and tell me which picture you think it is." (Have the child color the picture if he chooses correctly.)

1. This is something that grows outside.
   It may feel prickly or sticky.
   It doesn't make a sound.
   What is it? (evergreen tree)

2. You can smell it when it's cooking.
   It tastes salty.
   It goes pop, pop, pop.
   What is it? (popcorn)

3. This does not make a sound.
   It is as quiet as can be.
   It is white.
   It feels very cold.
   What is it? (snowflake)

4. This is something you can hang on your tree.
   Santa's reindeer may wear them.
   Some can make big sounds - - ding, dong!
   Some can make little sounds - - jingle, jingle!
   What is it? (bell)

5. This is an animal.
   He feels furry.
   His hooves make a sound.
   If he lands on your roof at Christmas
   You may hear - clippety, clop.
   What is it? (reindeer)

6. This is a person.
   He wears lots of red.
   He goes HO, HO, HO!
   Who is he? (Santa)

7. This feels very hot.
   It smells smoky.
   You can hear it go crackle, crackle.
   What is it? (fire)

Other Suggestions/Activities

- Use for following directions. Ex: "Color the reindeer brown."

66

Using Your Senses

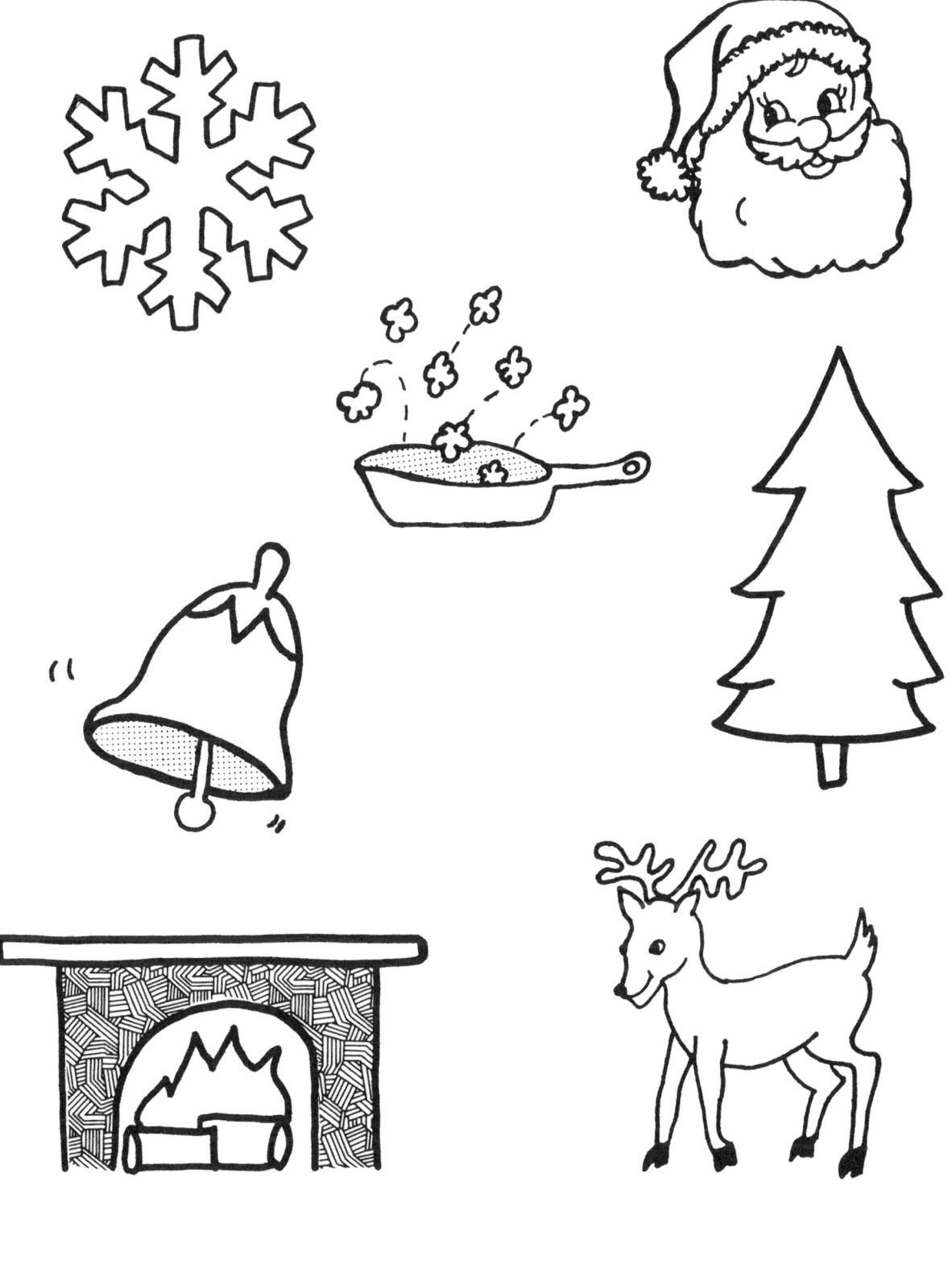

Name _____ Date _____

Christmas Story

Instructor: Read "A Special Christmas Tree" to child. If possible, use props to assist in attending skills. (Have a small tree nearby, a picture of Santa Claus, or wear a red cap like Santa.)

Storytime

Reproduce stick puppets (page 71). Have the child color, cut out, and paste on a tongue depressor or popsicle stick. Use while telling the story or have children hold up a stick puppet when they hear the name of their character in the story.

Other Suggestions/Activities

- Read one paragraph at a time and ask "WH" questions.

> Ex: Paragraph 1
> What is the weather like?
> Where do the girls live?
> What is mother going to bake?

- Have the child retell a part of the story using the stick puppets.

- Have the child draw a picture about the story and tell about the picture.

A Special Christmas Tree

Characters: Mother, Father, Ginny, Christine

It is a cold December morning on the farm. Ginny and Christine get up as the rooster crows. Mother, Father, and the girls are eating their breakfast. Mother says, "Today is December 24th, Christmas Eve. You need to finish your chores quickly. Then we can get ready for Christmas. I am baking banana nut bread today for your grandparents. We will give this to them on Christmas day."

"We have the special Christmas tree ornaments we made for Granny and PaPa," says Christine. "We want to remember people who are important to us at Christmas," says Ginny. "Yes, grand-parents are very special people," says Mother. Father says, "I want you girls to go with me today to cut down a Christmas tree. You can pick out our special tree this year."

Later that morning the girls are walking in the woods with Father. "There are so many trees. How can we choose?" asks Ginny. "Let's think of a plan," says Father. "We want an evergreen tree. Evergreens stay green all year. The trees that lose their leaves in cold weather are not used as Christmas trees. Our tree must be tall but not too tall. We need one that can stand up in the living room without touching the ceiling." "Let's remember that we want to have room for a star on top," says Christine.

Snow is starting to fall as they are looking for the tree. "Snowflakes look pretty on the trees," says Ginny. After looking carefully at many trees, the girls pick out a medium-sized evergreen tree. Father chops it down and they all help to carry it home.

After lunch, Father builds a fire in the fireplace. Mother hangs a wreath on the door. The girls are decorating the tree. They want ornaments and lights on the tree. They string popcorn with a needle and thread. "I love the smell of popcorn," says Ginny. "This will look so pretty on the Christmas tree. It makes me think about the snow-flakes on the trees outside," says Christine.

"What decorations should we put on first?" asks Ginny. "Let's put the lights on first," says Mother. "Second, we can put on the pop-corn strings," says Ginny. "Next, we put the pretty colored balls and other ornaments. Last, we put the star on the top," says Christine. "We will need to ask for Dad's help. He can hold me up so I can put the star on the very top," says Ginny.

The girls look out the window. "Look at all the snow. Do you think that Santa will have any trouble getting to our house?" asks Ginny. "Santa Claus wants to visit all the boys and girls tonight," says Mother. "His reindeer know all about traveling in snowy weather. They live in a very cold place. I am sure he is loading up his sleigh right now. He has a very long trip."

"We need to finish wrapping our presents," says Christine. "We need wrapping paper, tape, and ribbon." "We have our special ornaments for Granny and PaPa. We also have our presents for Mom and Dad," says Ginny. "It's important to remember giving to our family and friends," says Christine.

After supper, Ginny and Christine hang their stockings above the fire-place. Then they get ready for bed. Ginny is looking out the window at the snow. "Tomorrow we can ride our sled down the hill," says Ginny. "We can make a snowman, too," says Christine. "Let's make a real big one this year," says Ginny. "We can roll a very big snowball for the bottom, a medium snowball for the middle and a little one for his head." "He will need a hat and some gloves to keep warm," says Christine.

"We better go to sleep so Santa can come tonight. I wonder when he will be here," says Christine. "He has to visit all the boys and girls," says Ginny. "He is going to be very busy tonight. I hope he has time for the cookies and milk we left for him," says Christine. Ginny says, "I hope the reindeer eat the hay we left. They need to stop and rest, too!"

Christmas Story - Stick Puppets

<u>Instructions</u>: Have child color then cut out each character. Paste each character to the end of a tongue depressor or popsicle stick.

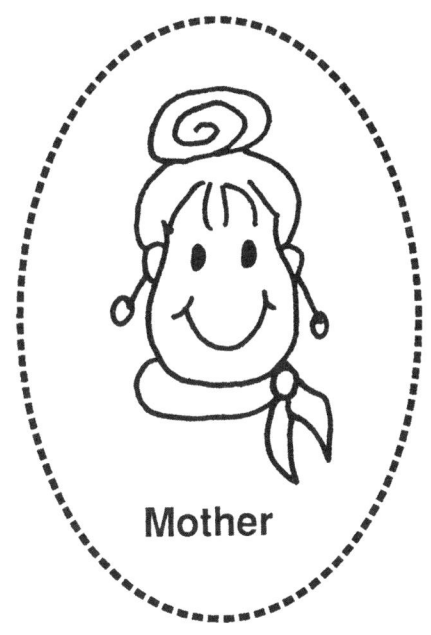

Mother

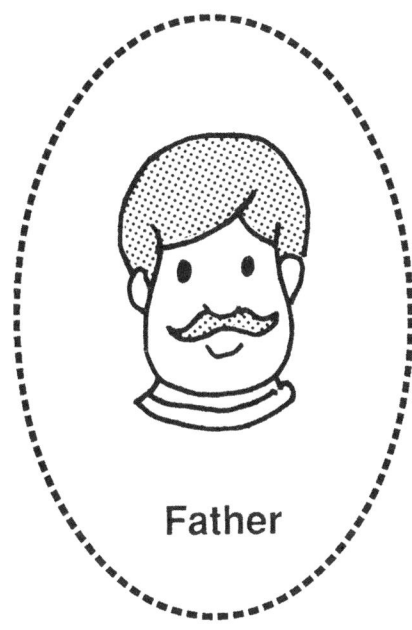

Father

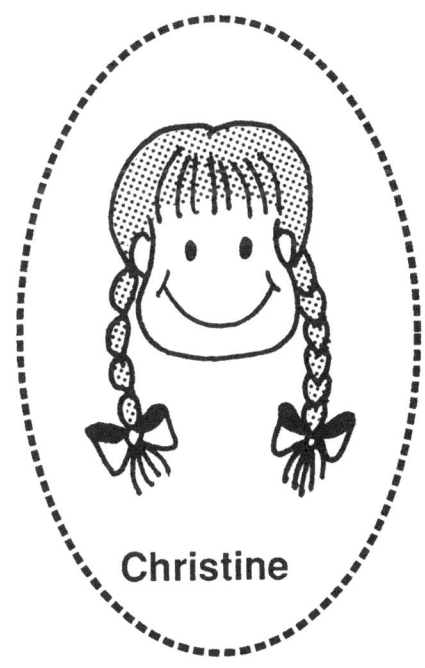

Christine

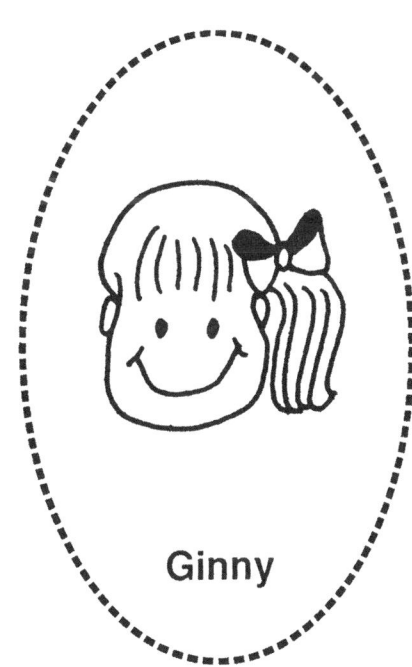

Ginny

Rhyming Time

Instructor: Reproduce stick puppets (page 73). Have the child color and cut out.
Paste each character to the end of a tongue depressor or popsicle stick.

Poem Time

Instructor: Read a poem. Have the children hold up a stick puppet when they hear
the name of their character.

Snowman

The Snowman doesn't
give two hoots,
He wears his hat-
But not his boots!

Santa

Santa is riding in his sleigh,
He has to go a long, long way.
In his sack are lots of toys.
For all the little girls and boys.

My Special Christmas Tree

The pretty snow is on the ground,
Evergreens are all around.
I'll pick one that's just for me,
To be my Special Christmas Tree.

Reindeer

I heard the bells in the night,
Jingle, Jingle - I was right!
I saw the reindeer in the sky,
I called out and said, "Goodbye."

Other Suggestions/Activities

- Sentence completion: Read a poem and leave off the last word in the line.
  Have the child complete the line by saying the word.

- Have the child learn one poem and recite it using a stick puppet.

- Rewrite a poem on large chart paper. Have the child draw a picture to go with
  the poem. Place on bulletin board.

Rhyming Time - Stick Puppets

Christmas - Worksheet 31

Instructions: Have child color then cut out each character. Paste each character to the end of a tongue depressor or popsicle stick.

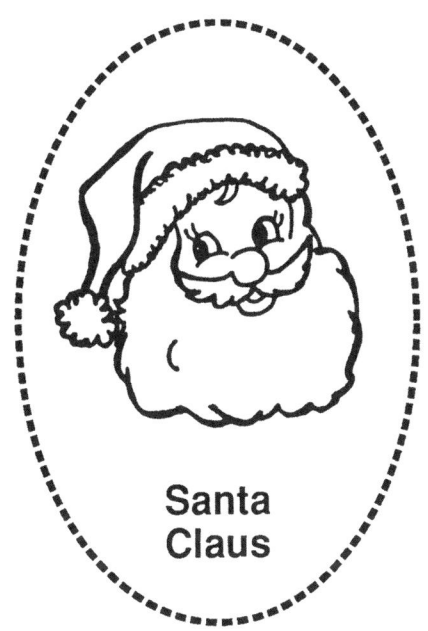

Santa Claus

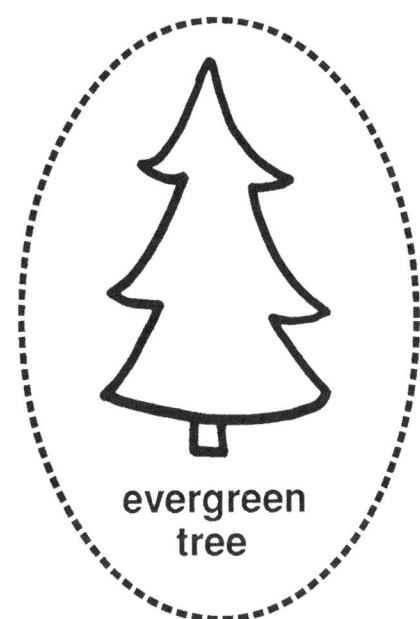

evergreen tree

snowman

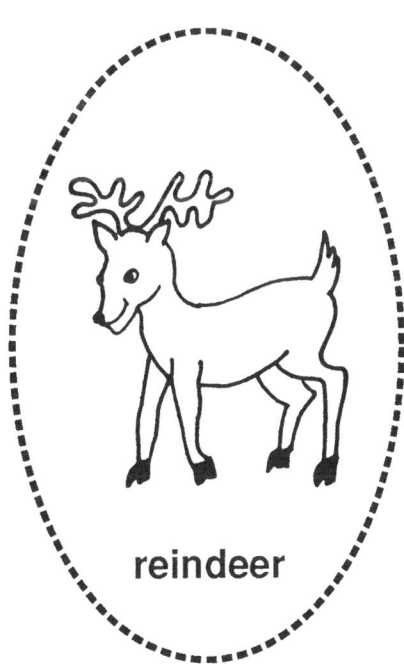

reindeer

73

Reindeer Time

Christmas - Worksheet 32

<u>Instructor</u>: Use patterns (page 75) and have child complete a paper bag reindeer puppet. For smaller children, parts can be pre-cut. Have child paste antlers, eyes, and nose on paper bag. Have the child tell about a reindeer.

Short Play

<u>Instructor</u>: Have children perform play.

Reindeer 1 -	"It's snowing outside."
Reindeer 2 -	"I hope we'll be able to see."
Reindeer 3 -	"Maybe we need flashlights."
Reindeer 4 -	"No, we will let Rudolph be first."

Have the children act out the following using the paper bag puppets.

One little reindeer is not enough,
Santa needs more because his job is tough.

Two little reindeers as fast as can be,
They'll do the job, just wait and see.

Three little reindeers, all ready to go,
Pulling the sleigh through the white, white snow.

Four little reindeers, up and away,
Can they pull that very big sleigh?

Five little reindeers, make it just right.
They help old Santa on Christmas Eve night.

Other Suggestions/Activities

- Model the sequence for making the reindeer puppet in group time. Place materials in center for child to make independently.

Reindeer Time

Christmas - Worksheet 32

Instructions: Use patterns below. Cut from colored construction paper. Have child paste parts on paper bag to make reindeer puppet.

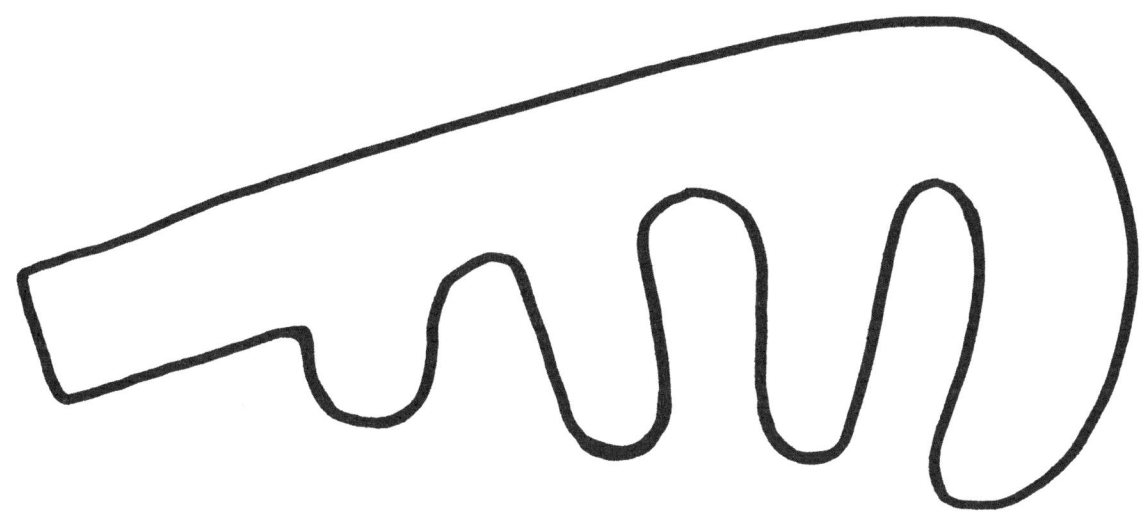

Brown antlers - Cut 2

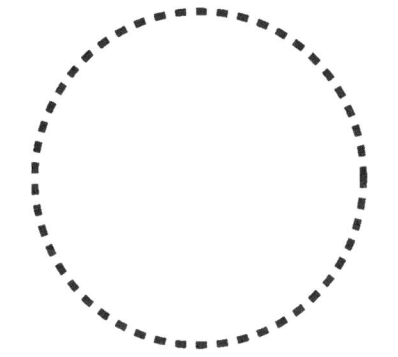

White outer eye - Cut 2

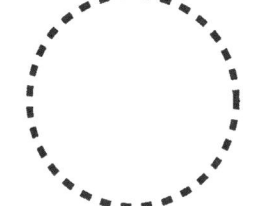

Black center of eye - Cut 2

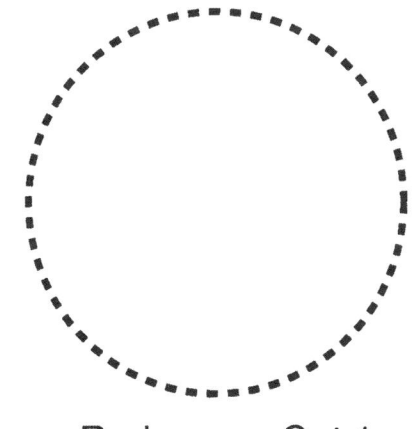

Red nose - Cut 1

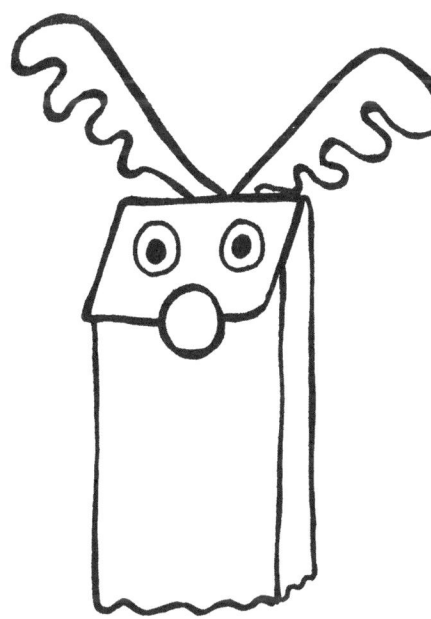

75

Christmas Game

Christmas - Worksheet 33

Instructor: Each child selects a marker, i.e. button or pawn. Flipping a penny can be used to determine movement. Ex: Heads - move ahead one space, Tails - move ahead two spaces.

Game Time

Reproduce one set of picture cards (pages 54 and 55). Have the child name the picture or tell one thing about the picture before he moves.

Other Suggestions/Activities

- Use the game board for the development of other vocabulary (i.e. colors, numbers, basic concept words.)

- Use in conjunction with riddles (page 56). Yes/no questions (page 64), or sentence completion (page 64). Have the child respond before moving.

- Use for unit review.

Santa is looking for his sleigh. Can you help him?

Christmas - Worksheet 33

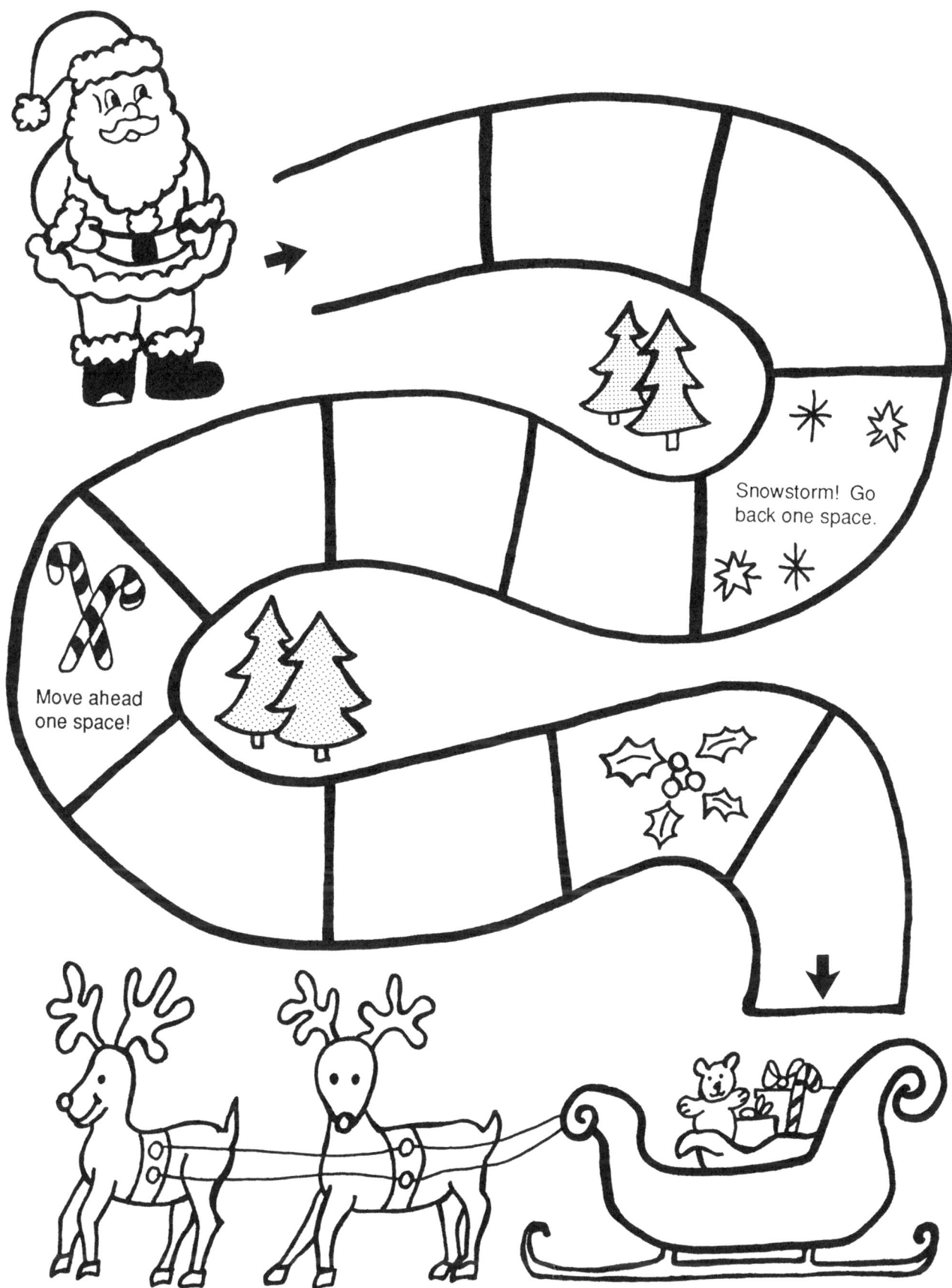

Snowstorm! Go back one space.

Move ahead one space!

Let's Talk About Hanukkah

Introduction to Hanukkah

Instructor: Tell the child about Hanukkah.

Ex: Hanukkah is a Jewish holiday that lasts eight days. The holiday begins on the 25th day of Kislev which is the third month of the Jewish calendar. Hanukkah means "dedication." Each day at sundown, a candle is lit on a menorah. A menorah is a special candle holder that holds eight candles and a helper candle that is used to light the others. Each night of Hanukkah, children receive gifts. Sometimes they are given coins. These are made of metal or sometimes chocolate. Another word for these coins is "gelt." A special food that is eaten during Hanukkah are potato pancakes and applesauce. Children may play with a special wooden top called a dreidel.

Core Vocabulary

Use the picture cards (page 79) to introduce the Hanukkah core vocabulary. Have the child color the pictures. The pictures may be cut out and mounted on light cardboard. Describe each picture. Tell about the size, color, or particular attributes of each object.

Match-up Activity

Reproduce two of each picture to make a set. Have the child find the matching pictures after you have scrambled them.

Memory Game

Place two to four cards on the table. Have the child look at the cards for a few seconds. Cover or turn them over. Have the child name the pictures from memory.

Other Suggestions/Activities

- Reproduce two of each picture. Use to play concentration game.

- Ask questions and have the child select the correct picture. Ex: Instructor says, "I am thinking of something good to eat during Hanukkah. What is it? " (potato pancakes)

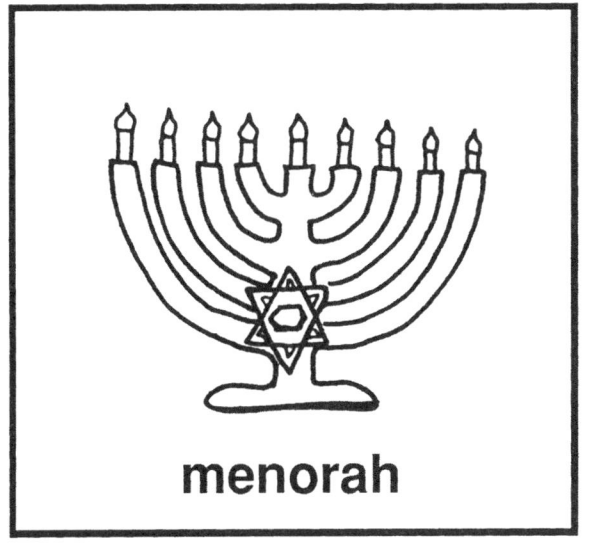

menorah

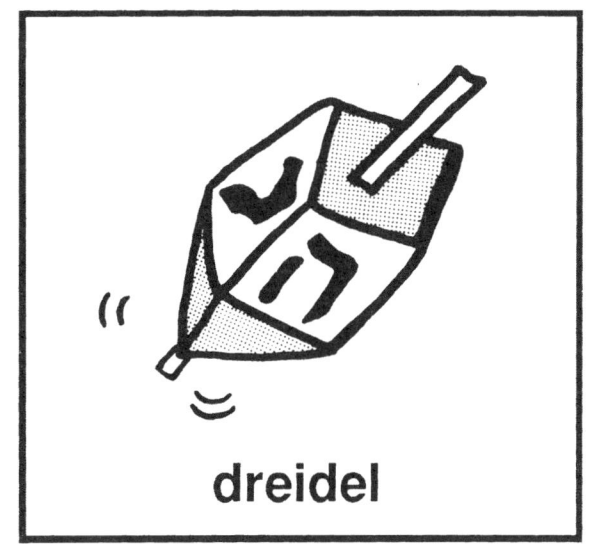

dreidel

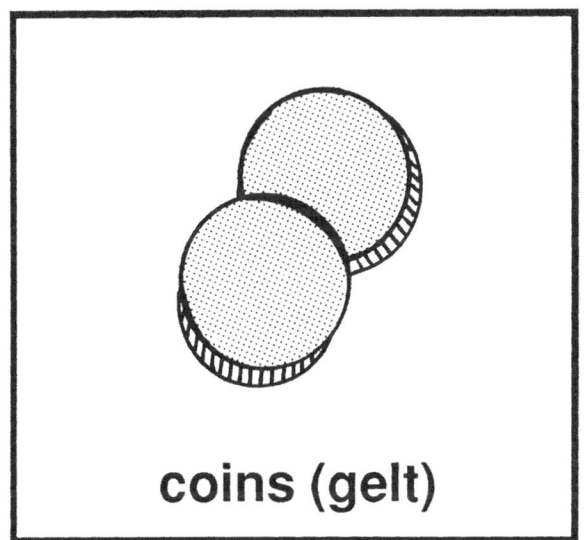

coins (gelt)

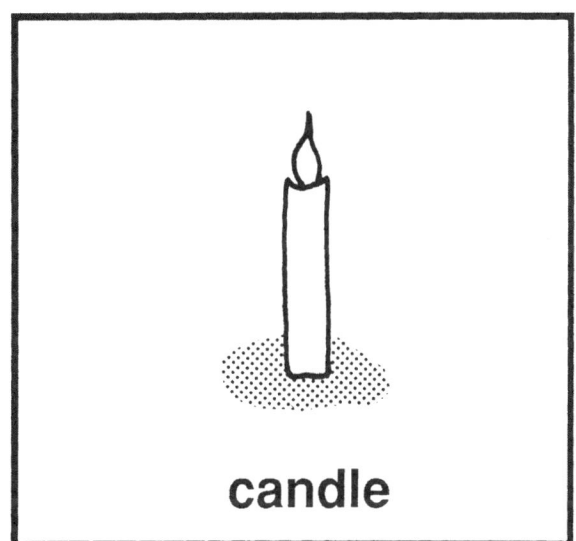

candle

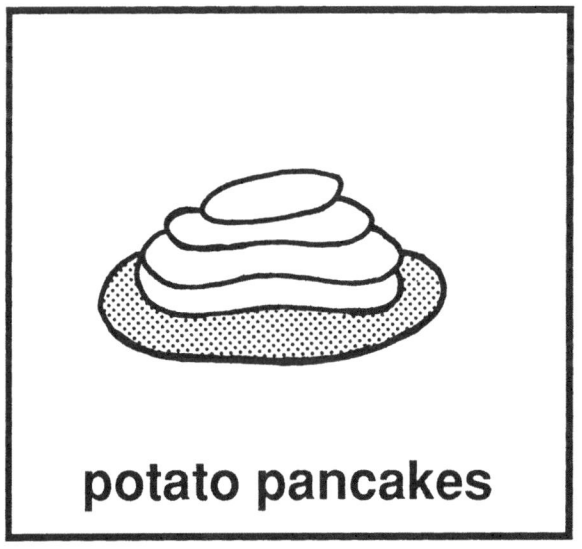

potato pancakes

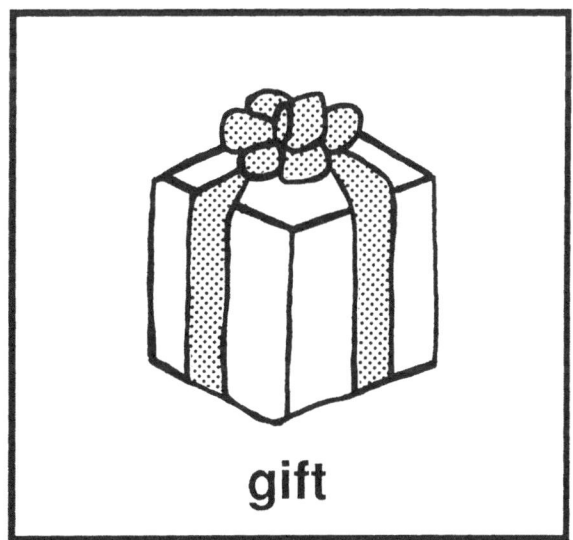

gift

Riddle Time

Instructor: Read each riddle below. Have the child choose which picture is being described. When the child chooses correctly, the picture can be colored.

1. It is a toy.
   It is a top.
   It is made of wood.
   It has letters on it.
   What is it? (dreidel)

2. It holds candles.
   It is used during Hanukkah.
   It holds eight candles and
    a helper candle.
   What is it? (menorah)

3. It is made of wax.
   You can put it in a
    special holder.
   You can light it.
   It has a wick.
   What is it? (candle)

4. It is wrapped with paper
    and has a pretty bow.
   You give it to other people.
   It has a surprise inside.
   What is it? (gift)

5. They are made of metal.
   They are shiny.
   They are round and flat.
   Children may get them
    during Hanukkah.
   What are they? (coins)

6. It is a food.
   They are eaten with applesauce.
   They are round and flat.
   They are made with potatoes.
   What are they? (potato pancakes)

Other Suggestions/Activities

- Have the child name each picture and color it.

- Have the child choose a picture and describe it or have the child make up
  his own riddle.

- Say a sentence and have the child listen for a key word, i.e. "The candle was
  burning in the night." When the child hears the word candle, he draws a circle
  around the candle.

80

Riddle Time

Hanukkah - Worksheet 35

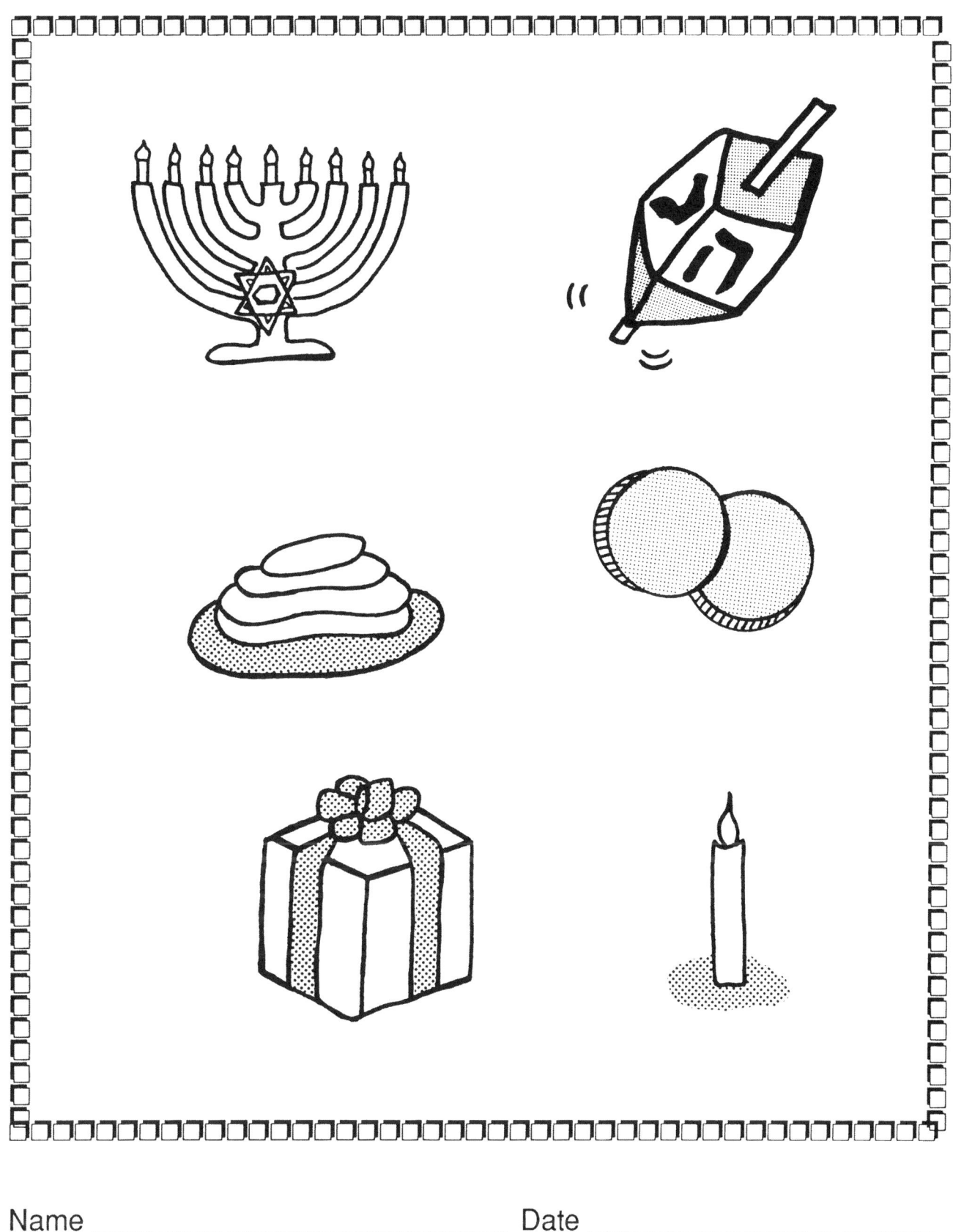

Name _____ Date _____

81

Eight Little Candles

Hanukkah - Worksheet 36

Instructor: "Listen carefully. I will tell you something. If I am right, answer YES. If I am wrong, answer NO." (When the child's response is correct he can paste a flame on the candle.)

1. A dreidel is a toy. (yes)
2. A menorah holds light bulbs. (no)
3. Hanukkah is a special holiday. (yes)
4. Coins are made of metal. (yes)
5. Potato pancakes are made of corn. (no)
6. You can eat applesauce with potato pancakes. (yes)
7. A candle is made of wax. (yes)
8. Hanukkah last two weeks. (no)

Sentence Completion

Instructor: "Listen carefully. I will say part of a sentence. When I stop, you say a word to finish the sentence." (When the child's response is correct, a flame can be pasted on the candle.)

1. A dreidel is a _____. (top, toy)
2. You put candles in a _____. (menorah)
3. Hanukkah is a Jewish _____. (holiday)
4. A surprise you give to someone else is a _____. (gift)
5. Coins are made of _____. (metal)
6. Potato pancakes are made from _____. (potatoes)
7. Potato pancakes can be eaten with _____. (applesauce)
8. Hanukkah lasts eight _____. (days)

Other Suggestions/Activities

- Number the flames 1-8. Have the child practice counting.

- Discuss a menorah. Have child color menorah and paste flames on candles. Hang picture on bulletin board.

Eight Little Candles

Hanukkah - Worksheet 36

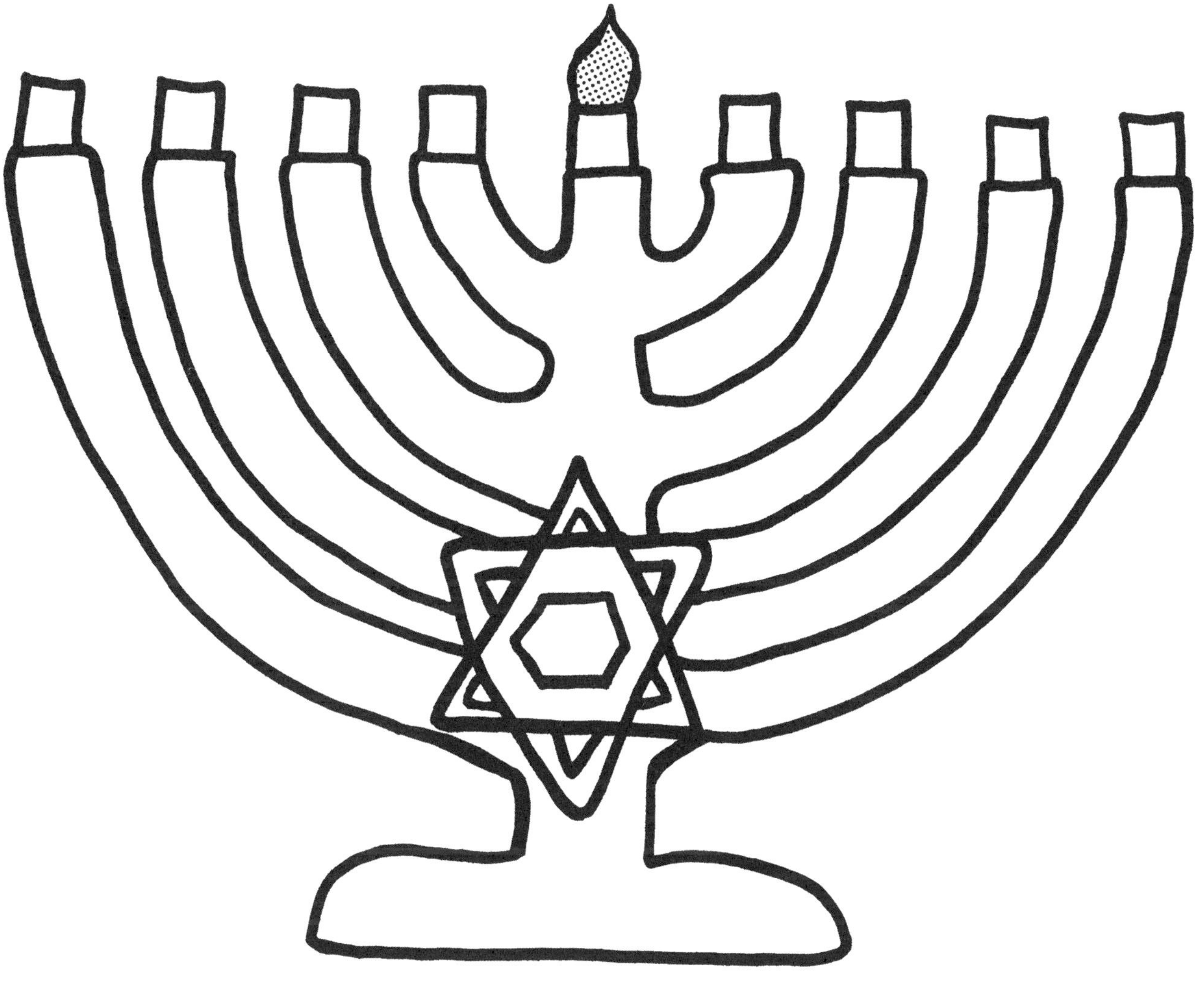

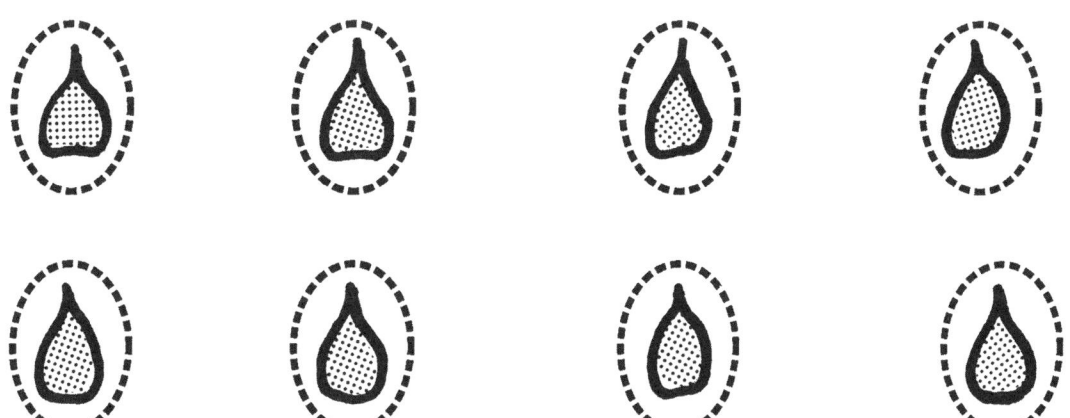

83

Hanukkah Story

Instructor: Read "A Day With Friends" to child. If possible use props to assist in attending skills. (Light a candle, play with a dreidel, or have potato pancakes to sample.)

Storytime

Reproduce stick puppets (page 87).   Have the child color, cut out, and paste on a tongue depressor or popsicle stick. Use while telling the story or have children hold up a stick puppet when they hear the name of their character in the story. Use the stick puppets and have the child retell a part of the story.

Other Suggestions/Activities

- Read one paragraph at a time and ask "WH" questions.

      Ex: Paragraph 1
           What kind of day is it?
           What is the boy's name?
           Where is he going?

- Have the child draw a picture about the story and tell about his picture.

A Day With Friends

Characters: Mother, David, Benjamin, Matt

One cold December day Matt is going out to play. "Mom, I'm going to David's house," says Matt. "Be careful crossing the street," says Mom.

When Matt gets to David's house, he sees David and his brother Benjamin playing a game with a small toy. "What are you playing?" asks Matt. "This is a top. It's called a dreidel," says David. "I don't have one of those. Tell me about it," says Matt. "This is a very old toy. Children have played with these for years and years," says Benjamin. "Sometimes our Granddad talks about playing with the dreidel when he was a small boy. The letters on the dreidel, stand for 'A Miracle Happened There,'" says David.

The children play a game with the dreidel. They laugh and have fun. David's mother is cooking in the kitchen. She talks to Matt about her special meal. "I am cooking potato pancakes. We call them potato latkes. We eat them for supper during our special holiday, Hanukkah. It's a tradition - like some people eat turkey at Thanksgiving. We eat potato pancakes and applesauce," says David's mother.

"I've never had potato pancakes. How do you make them?" asks Matt. "First, I cook potatoes. Next, I mix them with flour, eggs, and seasoning. Then I cook them on a skillet, just like your mom cooks pancakes. Last, we put applesauce on them," says David's mother.

"Tell me more about your special holiday," says Matt. David, Benjamin, and their mother are talking with Matt. "Hanukkah is a special holiday. It is the Jewish Feast of Lights. Hanukkah means 'dedication.' It begins on the twenty-fifth day of the Jewish month of Kislev. This comes in December. It lasts eight days," says Mother. "Each day we light a new candle on the menorah," says David. "What's a menorah?" asks Matt. "A menorah is a special candle holder with eight candles and a helper candle in the center. The center one is used to light each new candle at sundown," says Benjamin.

"Tell me more about Hanukkah," says Matt. "Each night of Hanukkah, the children get a gift," says David. "The children are also given coins.

These are called 'gelt.' Sometimes the coins are made of metal and sometimes they are made of chocolate! Hanukkah is a happy time," says Benjamin.

"Thank you for sharing with me," says Matt. "We like to teach others about our Jewish traditions. When we listen and learn about other people's traditions, we learn to respect those traditions," says Mother.

"Every year Mom comes to school and makes potato pancakes during Hanukkah," says David. "What do the kids say about that?" asks Matt. David and Benjamin smile and say, "YUM! YUM!"

Hanukkah Story - Stick Puppets

Hanukkah - Worsheet 37

<u>Instructions</u>: Have child color then cut out each character. Paste each character to the
end of a tongue depressor or popsicle stick.

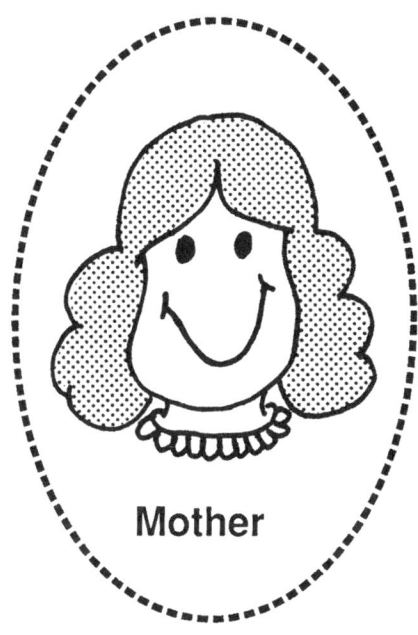

Mother

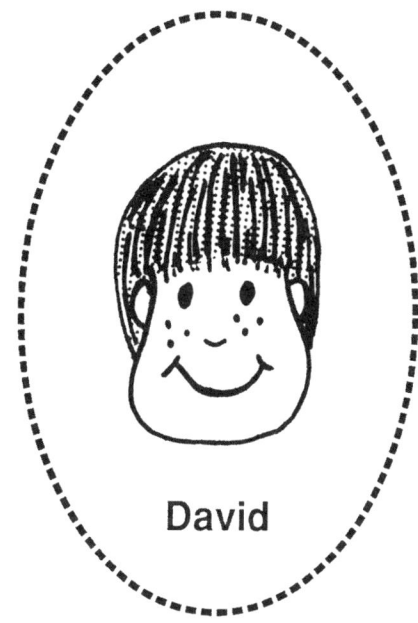

David

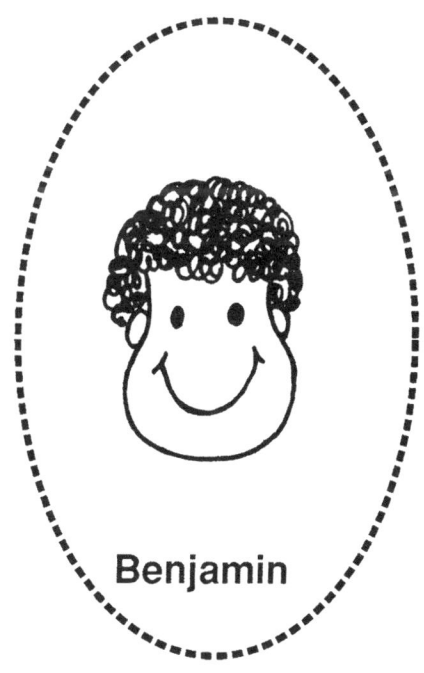

Benjamin

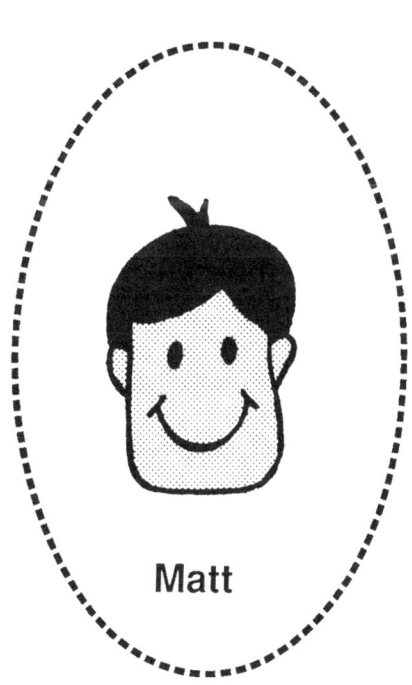

Matt

87

Rhyming Time

Instructor: Reproduce stick puppets (page 89). Have child color and cut out.
Paste each figure to the end of a tongue depressor or popsicle stick.

Poem Time

Menorah

The candles are glowing,
In the night.
Eight candles burning,
Very bright.

Dreidel

The dreidel is a toy.
A tiny wooden top.
Letters on the outside.
It will spin and stop.

Gelt

Coins children get,
at Hanukkah time.
Some made of chocolate
and tasting so fine!

Hanukkah

Hanukkah is a holiday.
It is the feast of lights.
We celebrate in a special way,
It lasts eight bright nights.

Potato Pancakes

Potato pancakes are very nice,
My mother makes them once or twice.
I like to eat them late at night,
With applesauce - they are just right.

Instructor: Have the child complete a stick puppet on page 89. Have the child draw a
a picture to go with the poem. Place on bulletin board.

Other Suggestions/Activities

- Rewrite a poem on large chart paper. Have the child draw a picture to go with the
  poem. Place on bulletin board.

- Sentence completion: Read a poem and leave off the last word in the line. Have
  the child complete the line by saying the word.

Rhyming Time - Stick Puppets

Hannukah - Worksheet 38

Instructions: Have child color then cut out each character. Paste each character to the end of a tongue depressor or popsicle stick.

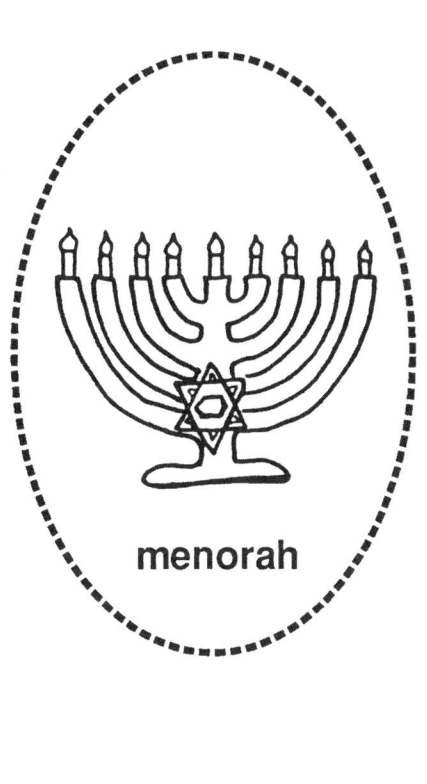

menorah

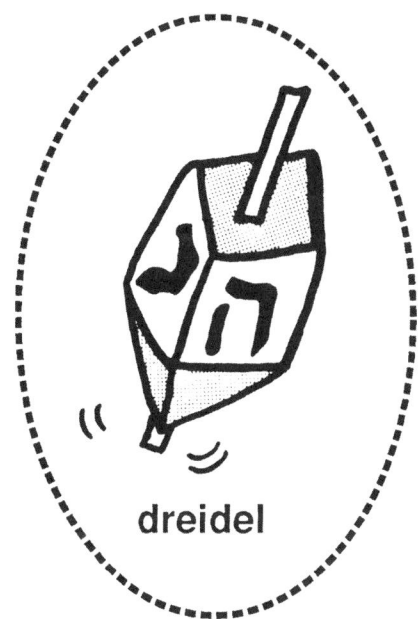

dreidel

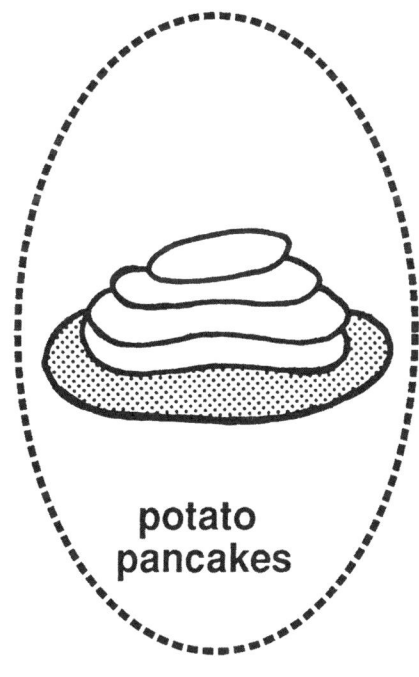

potato pancakes

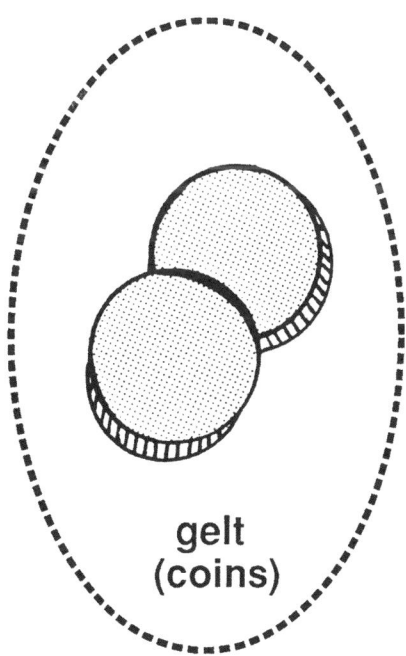

gelt (coins)

Hanukkah Game

Instructor: Each child selects a marker, i.e. button or pawn. Flipping a penny can be used to determine movement. Ex: Heads - move ahead one space, Tails - move ahead two spaces.

Reproduce one set of picture cards (page 79). Have the child name the picture or tell one thing about the picture before he moves.

Other Suggestions/Activities

- Use the gameboard for the development of other vocabulary. (i.e. colors, numbers, basic concept words)

- Use in conjunction with riddles (page 88), yes/no questions (page 82), or sentence completion (page 82). Have the child respond before moving.

- Use for unit review.

David is looking for his dreidel. Help him find it!

Hanukkah - Worksheet 39

Found some gelt.
Move ahead one
space!

Stopped to eat potato pancakes.
Go back one space.

91

Let's Talk About Valentine's Day

Valentine's Day - Worksheet 40

Introduction to Valentine's Day

Instructor: Tell the child about Valentine's Day.

Ex: Valentine's Day is February 14th. On Valentine's Day, we show love to our family and friends by sending them special cards, flowers, or candy. At school we may make our own valentines. We may have a special box that we decorate for our friends to put our valentines in.

We can send valentines to others in the mail. We have to remember to put the other person's address on the envelope. We also put our address in one corner and a stamp in the other corner. The mail carrier will take our valentine to the main post office. At the main post office another mail carrier will take our valentine to the person. If the person lives far away, our valentine might go by airplane or truck to the city where they live.

Core Vocabulary

Use the picture cards (pages 94 and 95) to introduce the Valentine core vocabulary. Have the child color the pictures. The pictures may be cut out and mounted on light cardboard. Describe each picture. Tell about the size, color, or particular attributes of each object.

Match-up Activity

Reproduce two of each picture to make a set. Have the child find the matching pictures after you have scrambled them.

Memory Game

Place two to four cards on the table. Have the child look at the cards for a few seconds. Cover or turn them over. Have the child name the pictures from memory.

Other Suggestions/Activities

- Reproduce two of each picture. Use to play concentration game.

- Have a brainstorming time. Ex: Instructor chooses the mailbox picture card. Ask the child to name all the things that could fit in a mailbox. Encourage the child to use his imagination (light bulb, turtle, doughnut, socks, pencil, etc.) Now ask the child to name things that could not fit in the mail box!

Use the brainstorming technique on each picture card.

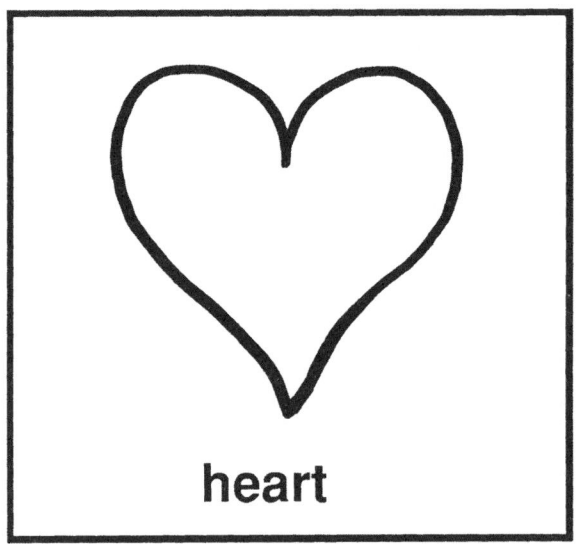

heart

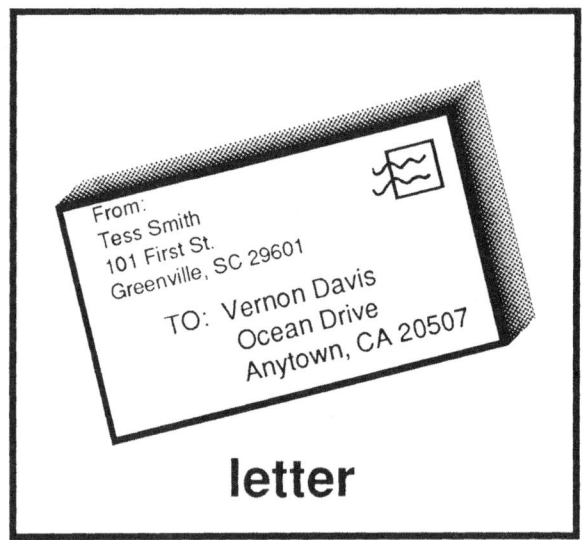

letter

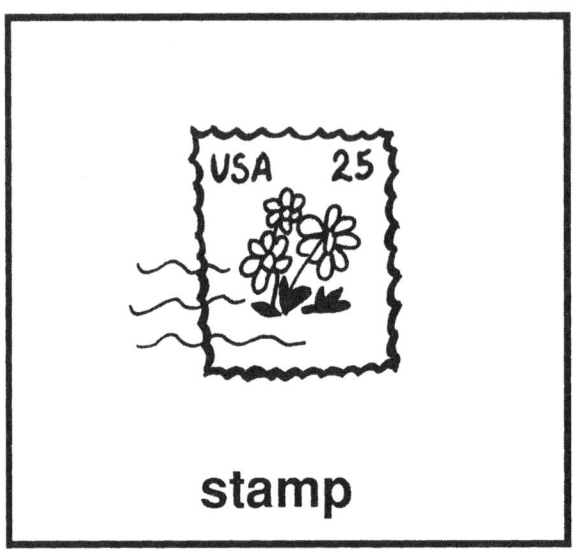

stamp

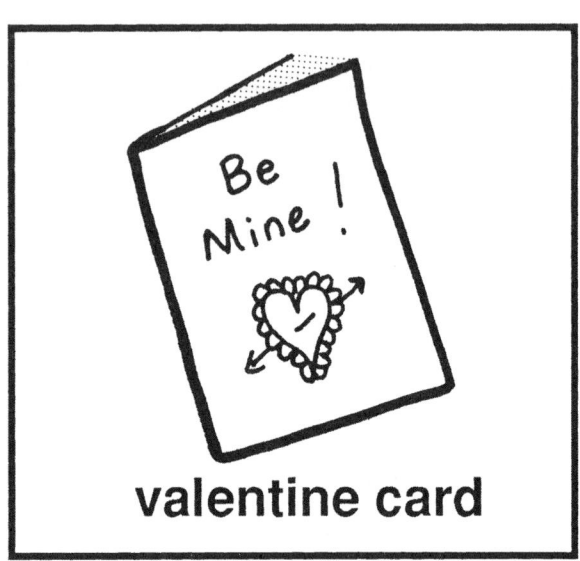

valentine card

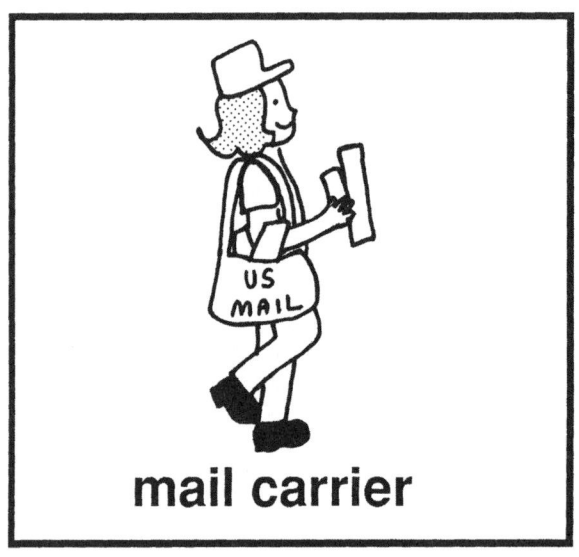

mail carrier

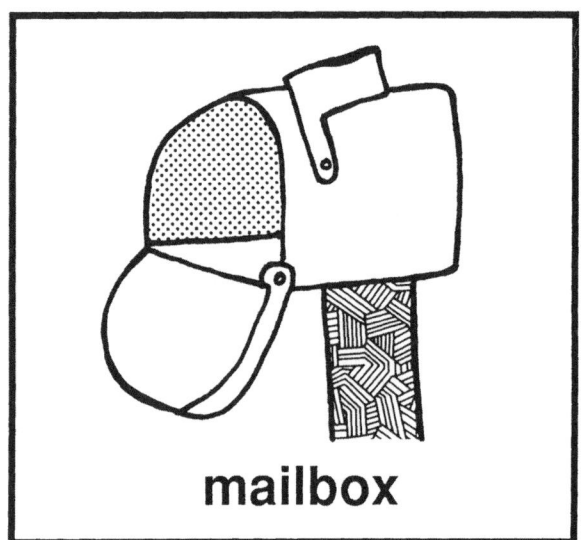

mailbox

94

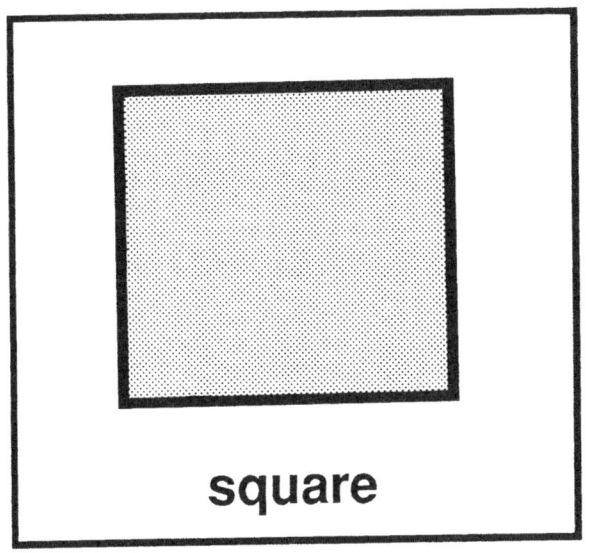

square

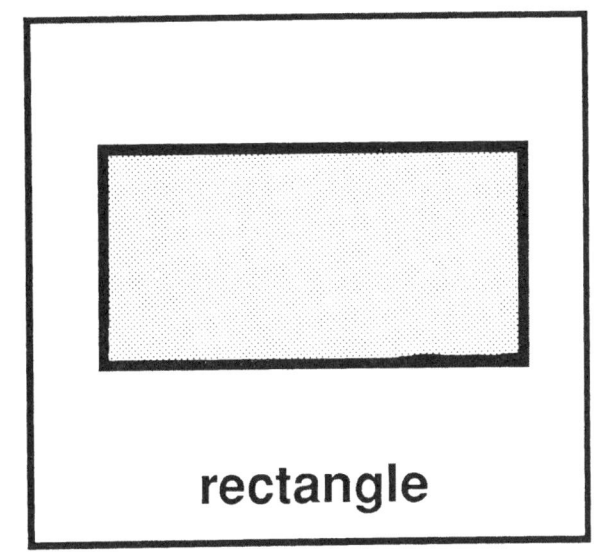

rectangle

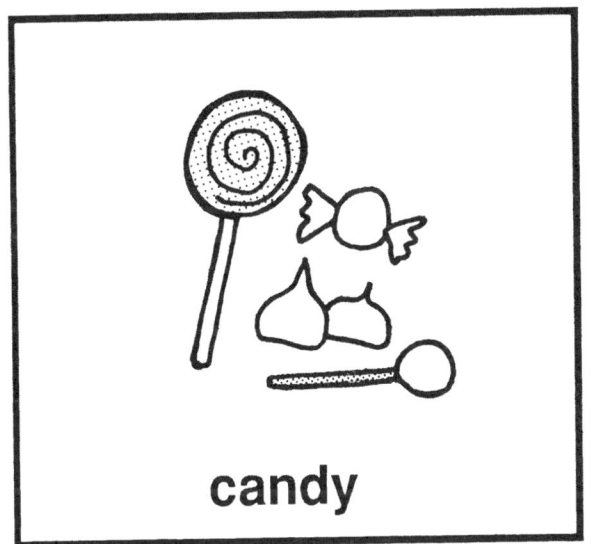

candy

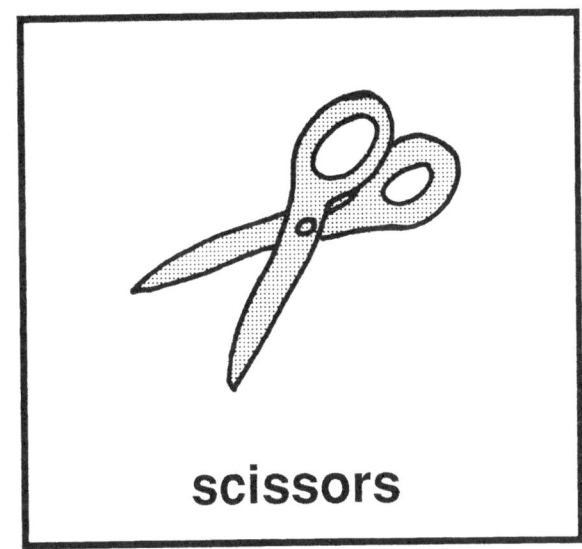

scissors

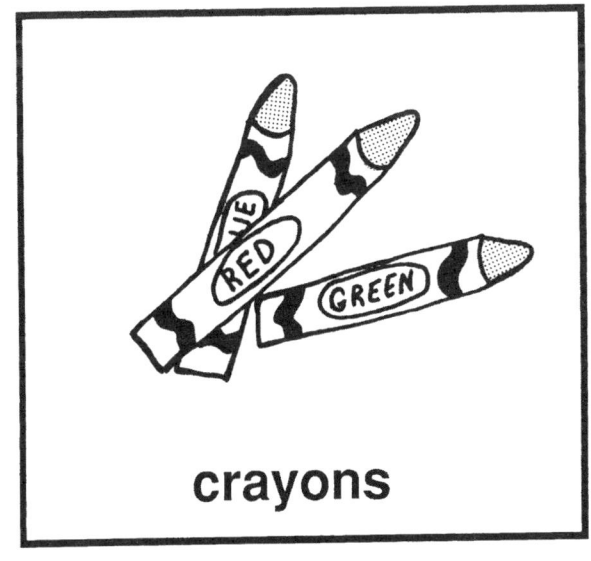

crayons

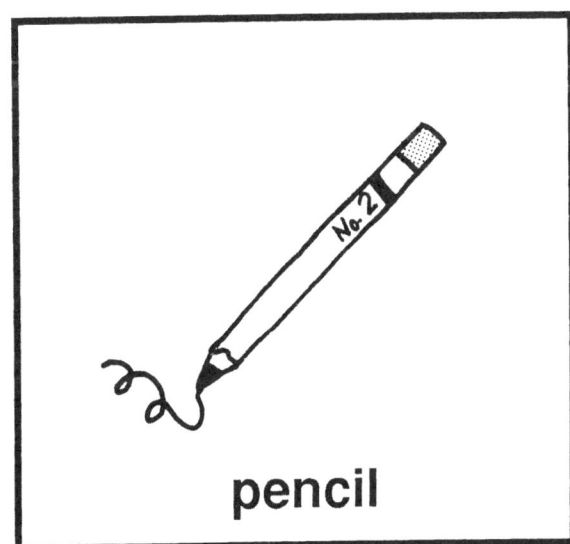

pencil

Riddle Time

Instructor: Read each riddle below. Have the child choose which picture is being described. When the child chooses correctly, the picture can be colored.

1. It is a shape.
   It has curved lines at the top.
   It comes to a point at the bottom.
   It can be red or pink.
   It is seen on a Valentine card.
   What is it? (heart)

2. It is made of paper.
   We send it to someone.
   It has their address on it.
   It has a stamp on it.
   We put a message inside.
   The mail carrier delivers it.
   What is it? (letter)

3. It is made of paper.
   It is small.
   It has glue on the back.
   We lick it and put it on a letter.
   What is it? (stamp)

4. It is made of paper.
   We give it to someone on
      Valentine's Day.
   We sign our name on the back.
   It has hearts and words on it.
   It can say, "I love you" or
      "Be my friend."
   What is it? (Valentine card)

5. It is a person.
   He/she wears a uniform.
   He/she can drive a truck
      or can walk.
   He/she delivers our letters
      and cards.
   Who is it? (mail carrier)

6. It is made of metal.
   It holds letters, cards, or
      small packages.
   It can be on our house or
      out by our street.
   What is it? (mailbox)

7. It is a shape.
   It has 4 corners.
   It has 4 sides.
   All sides are the same length.
   What is it? (square)

8. It is a shape.
   It has 4 corners.
   It has 4 sides.
   Two sides are long.
   Two sides are short.
   What is it? (rectangle)

9. It is something to eat.
   It tastes sweet.
   It is made with sugar.
   What is it? (candy)

10. These are made of
       metal or plastic.
    They have handles.
    We use these to cut paper.
    What are they? (scissors)

11. It is long and skinny.
    It is made of wood.
    It has lead on the inside.
    It has an eraser on one end.
    We write with it.
    What is it? (pencil)

12. These are made of
       colored wax.
    They have paper on
       the outside.
    We can draw with them.
    They can be red, yellow,
       blue, or green.
    What are they? (crayons)

Other Suggestions/Activities

- Have the child name each picture and color it.

- Have the child choose a picture and describe it or have the child make up his own riddle.

- Say a sentence and have the child listen for a key word, i.e. "I wrote a <u>letter</u> to my friend." When the child hears the word letter, he draws a circle around the picture.

Riddle Time

Valentine's Day - Worksheet 41

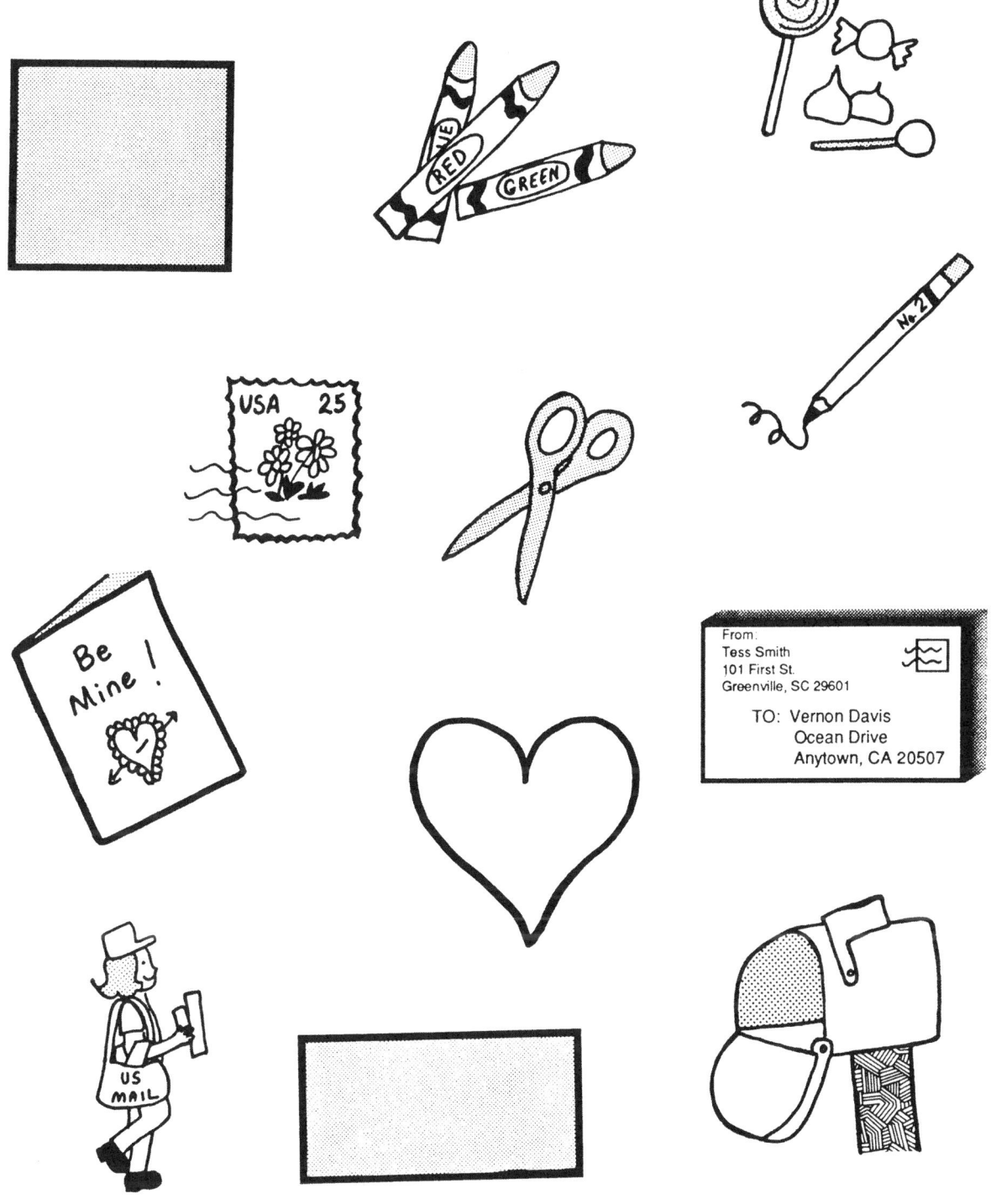

Name _____ Date _____

Shapes Match-Up

Valentine's Day - Worksheet 42

<u>**Instructor**</u>:   Reproduce one set of shapes. Cut apart and use for matching.

Discuss shapes with child. Have the child find objects in the room that have the same shape as the pictures on the worksheet.

Other Suggestions/Activities

- Reproduce the worksheet for each child. Have the child draw a line to match the shapes.

98

© 1999, Super Duper ® Publications

Shapes Match-Up

Valentine's Day - Worksheet 42

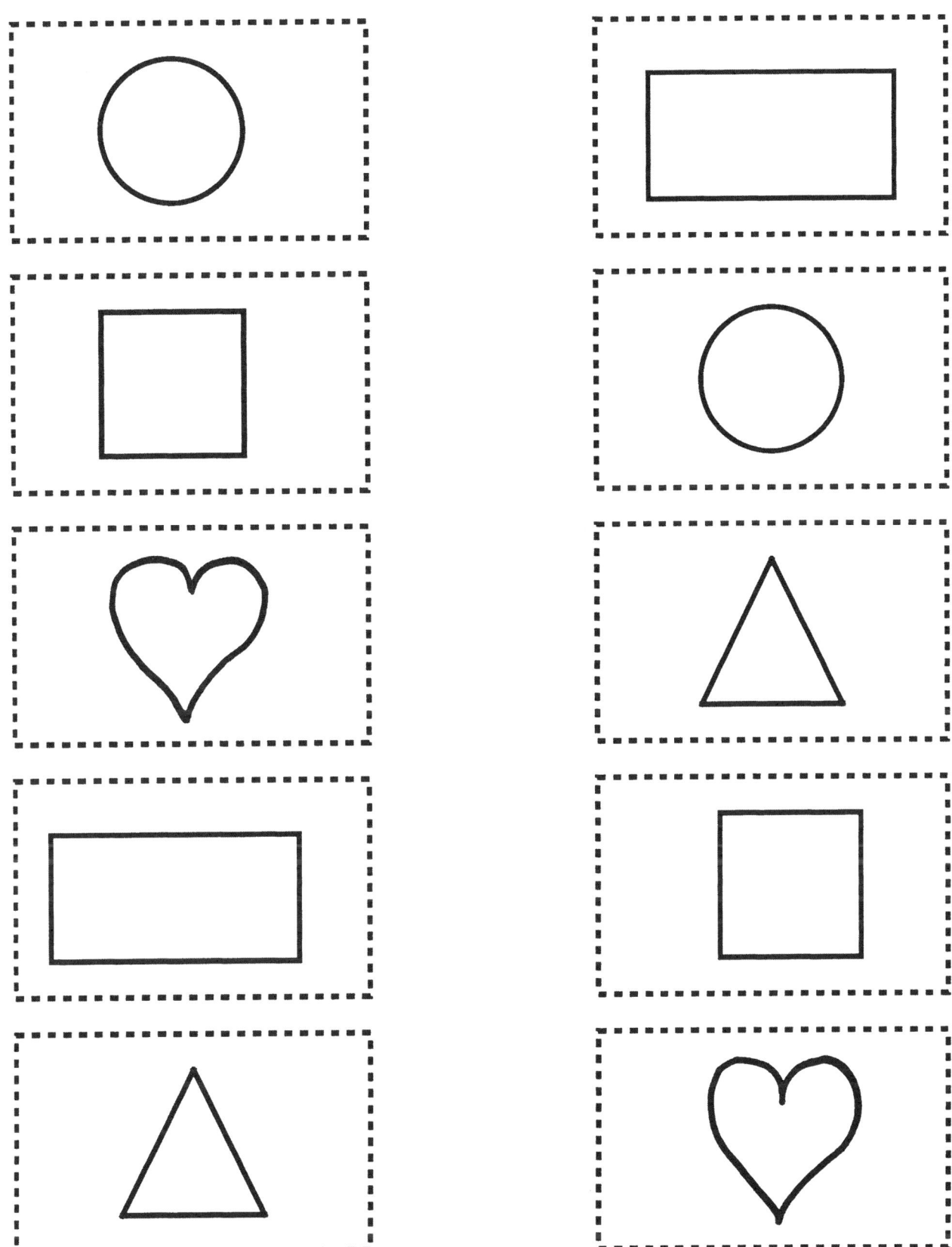

99

What's Hiding?

Valentine's Day - Worksheet 43

Instructor: "Listen carefully. I will ask you a question." (When the child's response is correct, a part of the picture can be colored.)

1. What date is Valentine's Day? (February 14)
2. Who delivers mail? (mail carrier)
3. What do we give people on Valentine's Day? (card)
4. What do we write on the front of a letter? (address)
5. What do we put mail in? (mailbox)
6. Where do we put a stamp? (on a letter, in the corner)
7. What shape has four sides that are all the same length? (square)
8. What do we use to cut with? (scissors)
9. What do we use to color with? (crayons, colors)
10. What do we use to write with? (pencil)
11. What can we eat that tastes sweet and is made with sugar? (candy)
12. What shape has two long sides and two shorter sides? (rectangle)

Other Suggestions/Activities

- Read the child a story about Valentine's Day. Discuss and ask questions.

- Have the child color the page and place on bulletin board.

What is hiding?

Valentine's Day - Worksheet 43

Color the R spaces red and the G spaces green.
What do you see?

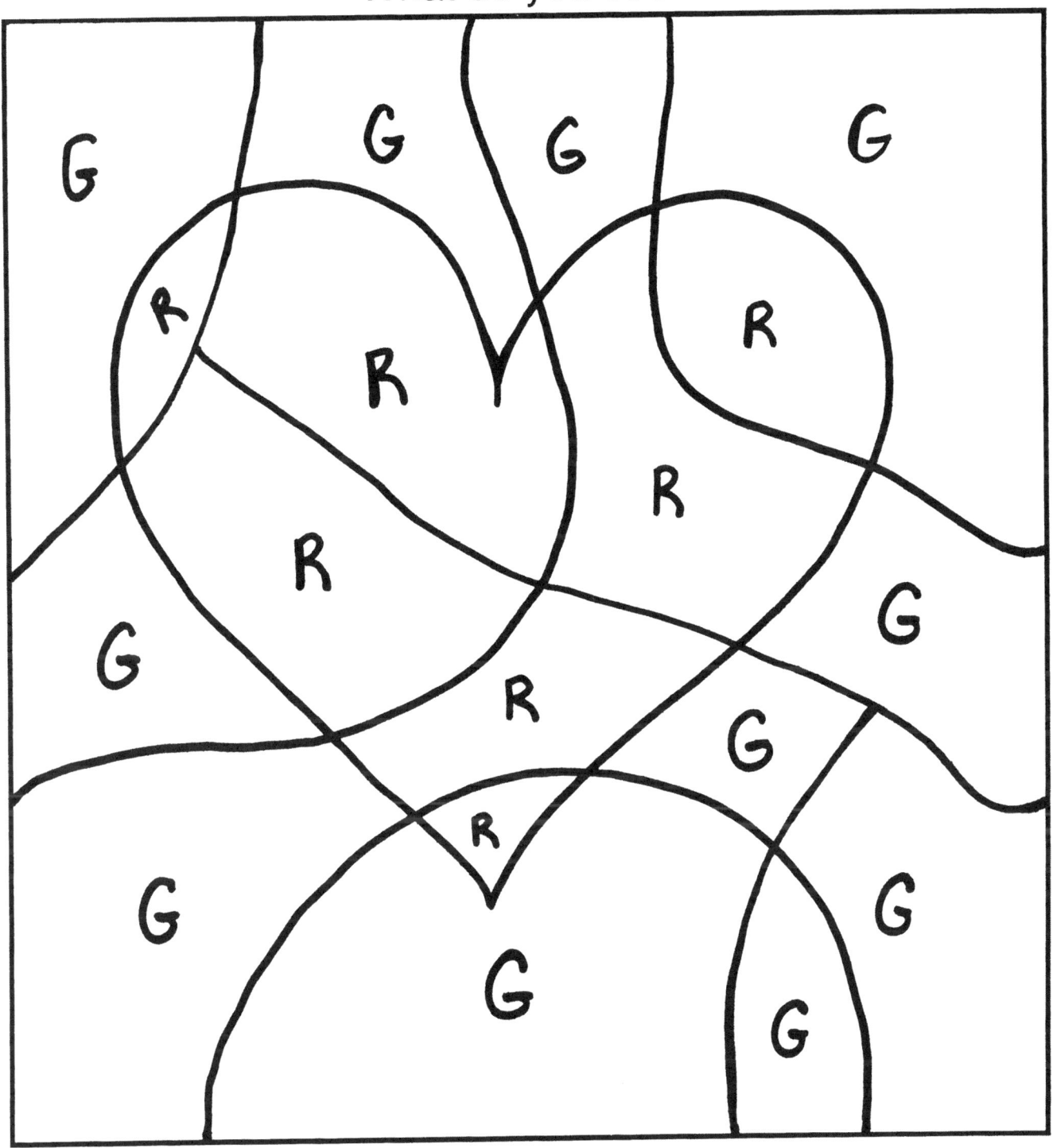

Name _____ Date _____

What's Your Address?

Instructor: Assist child in learning his address. Have child color the house and write his name and address at the bottom. Place on bulletin board.

Other Suggestions/Activities

- Have the child practice writing his address by writing a letter or sending a Valentine to his own house.

- Take a field trip to the post office. Have the child mail his own letter or card.

- Have the child bring to class the letter or card he mailed. Discuss how long it took, how it looks different (cancelled stamp, etc.)

- Make a bulletin board with letters and cards from different people from different places.

What's Your Address?

Valentine's Day - Worksheet 44

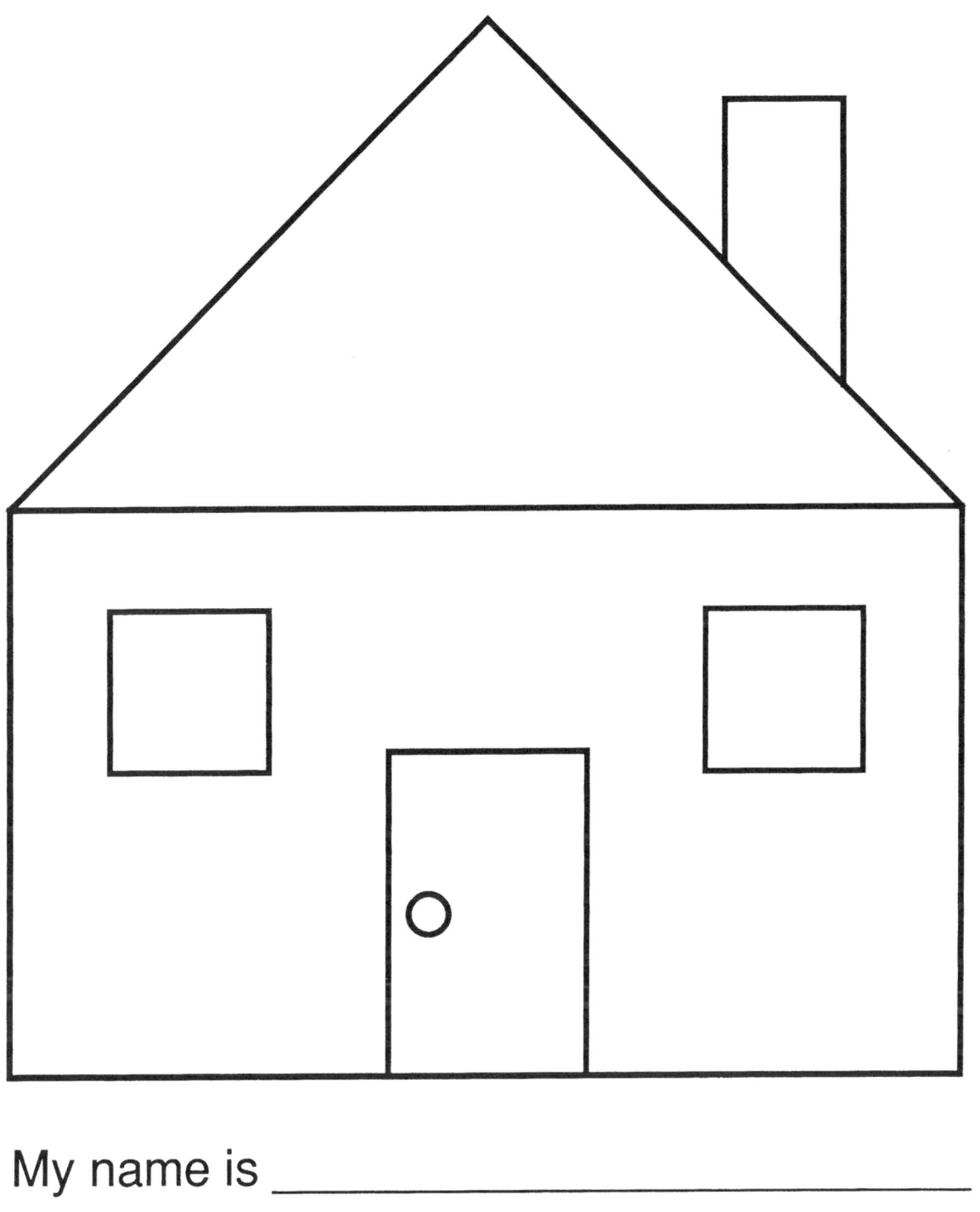

My name is _____

My address is _____

City _____ State _____

Zip code _____ Phone (_____) _____

Mail Truck
Valentine's Day - Worksheet 45

Instructor: Reproduce one copy of worksheet for each child. Have the child color, paste on light tagboard, and cut out.

Cut the top off a 1/2 pint milk carton. Have the child paste a mail truck to each side of the milk carton.

Mail Time

Discuss how mail travels. Some mail carriers walk. Some drive trucks. Find out from the child how mail is delivered in his neighborhood.

Other Suggestions/Activities

- Place mail trucks in play centers.

- For older children, place a U.S. map on the floor. Have the child "move mail" from two cities identifying the states along the way.

cut top off here

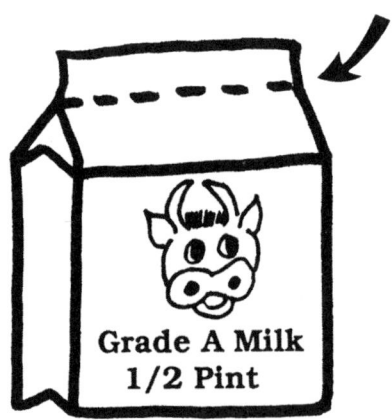

Grade A Milk
1/2 Pint

104

Mail Truck

Valentine's Day - Worksheet 45

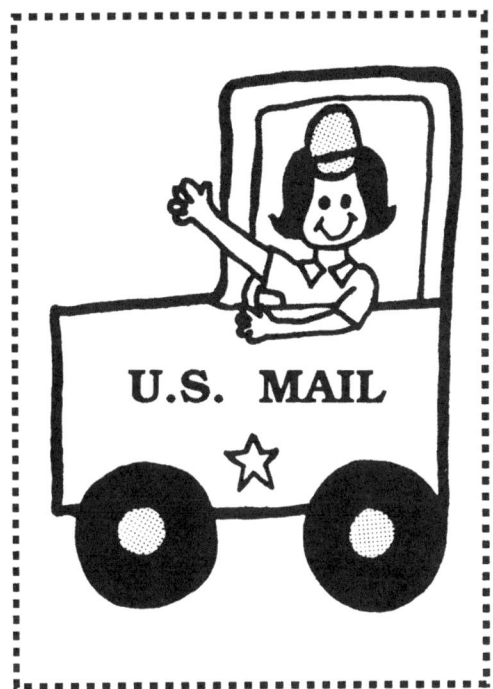

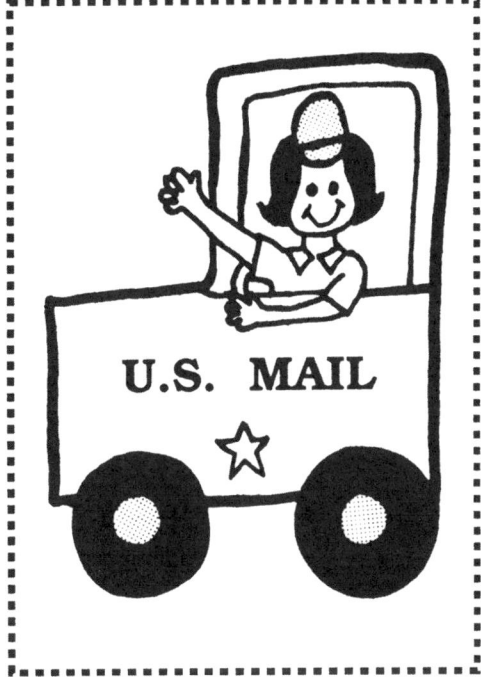

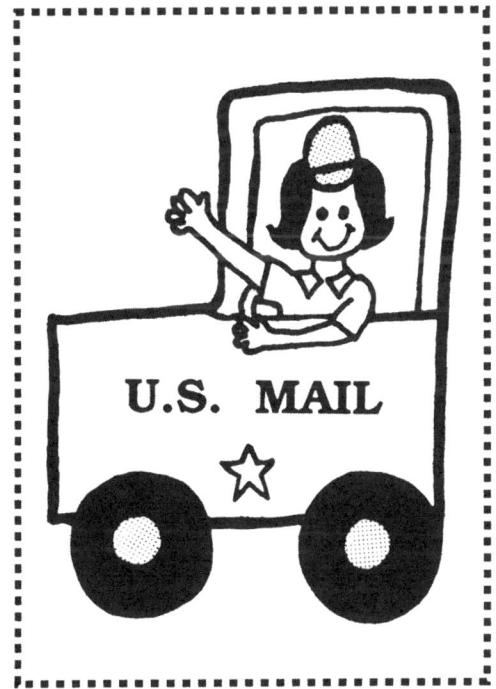

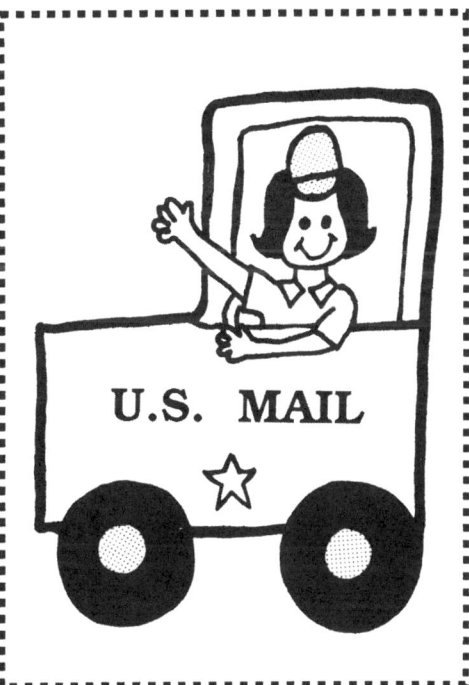

Lots of Hearts

Instructor: Have the child color and cut out the hearts on page 107. Paste on a paper bag or shoe box for a "Valentine Mailbox" to use in the classroom.

Other Suggestions/Activities

- Use the blank hearts for the child to write his own Valentine messages to his family and friends.

- Use an 8 1/2 x 11 sheet of white construction paper. Fold to make a Valentine card. Have the child use the hearts to make his own Valentine card.

Lots of Hearts

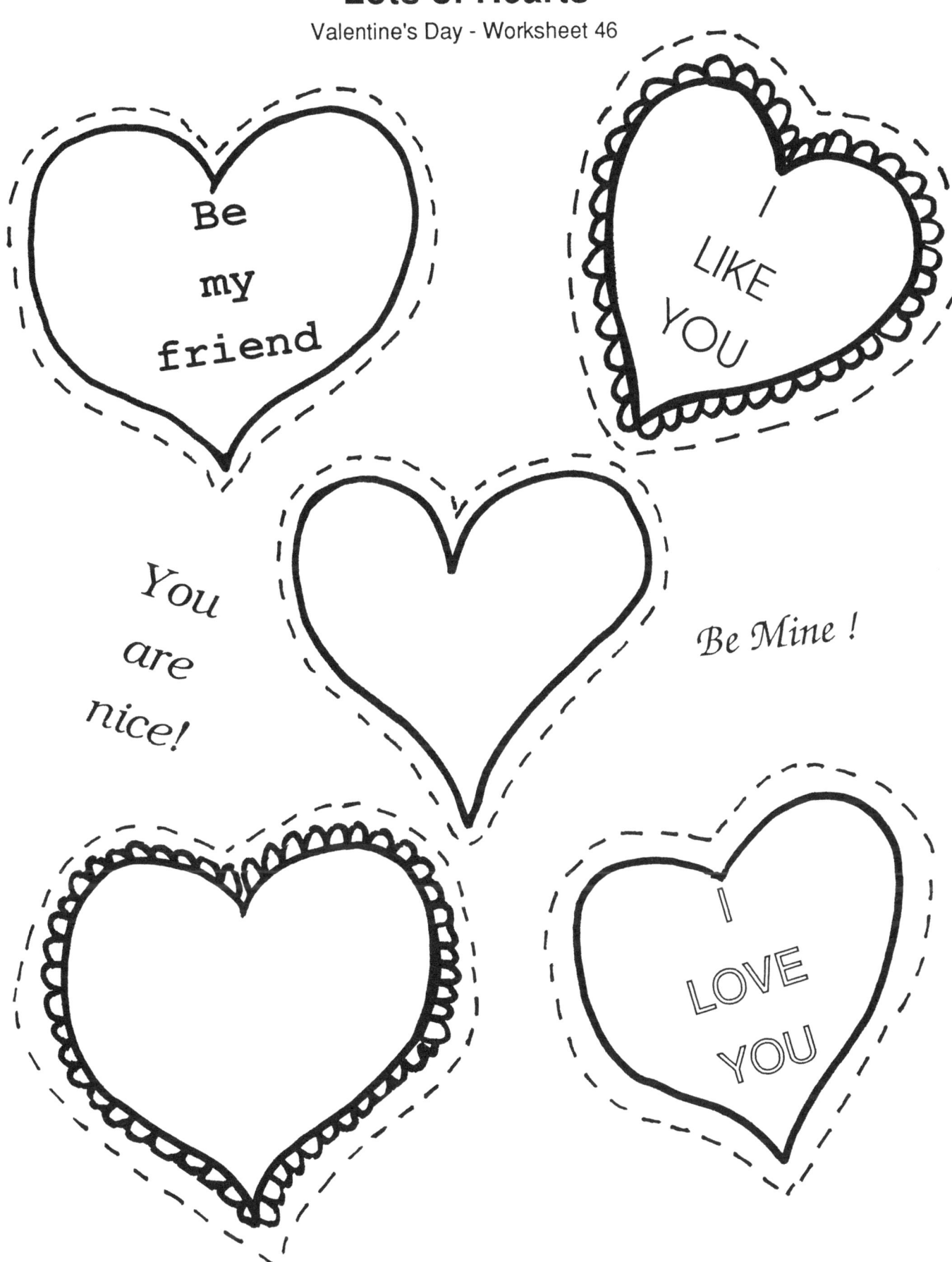

Be
my
friend

I
LIKE
YOU

You
are
nice!

Be Mine !

I
LOVE
YOU

107

Valentine's Day Story

Instructor: Read "Rosa's Valentines" to child. If possible, use props to assist in attending skills. (Have a big red heart, candy hearts, or a Valentine mailbox nearby.)

Storytime

Reproduce stick puppets (page 111). Have the child color, cut out, and paste on a tongue depressor or popsicle stick. Use while telling the story or have children hold up a stick puppet when they hear the name of their character in the story.

Use the stick puppets and have the child retell a part of the story.

Other Suggestions/Activities

- Read one paragraph at a time and ask "WH" questions.

        Ex: Paragraph 1
                What is the girl's name?
                What did she do when she got up?
                What day was it?

- Have the child draw a picture about the story and tell about his picture.

- The dog in the story does not have a name. Have a "Name Rosa's Dog" contest.
  Have children think of names for the dog. Vote to see which name is the favorite.

Rosa's Valentines

Characters: Rosa, Aunt Maria, Eunice, puppy

Rosa gets up early on Saturday morning. She watches cartoons while she eats breakfast. "I like Saturdays!" says Rosa to her puppy. "I can take my time. I don't like having to hear 'hurry up' every day. I need to have some time for you," Rosa tells her puppy. The puppy licks Rosa's hand. "I need to think of a name for you. We have so much fun together. We run and play chase. You follow me everywhere," says Rosa. The puppy wags his tail as Rosa pats him on the head.

After her favorite cartoons are over Rosa talks to her Aunt Maria. "I wish I could do something special today," says Rosa. "Well, let me think," says Aunt Maria. "There is a special day in February. It is a time to show love to our family and friends. We send special cards and letters. That day is February 14," says Aunt Maria.

"I know," says Rosa, "it's Valentine's Day!" "Let's send a special letter to Granny," says Aunt Maria. "I'll draw a picture for Granny," says Rosa. "I'll write her a note and we'll mail them to her," says Aunt Maria.

Later, Rosa and Aunt Maria are putting their letters in the envelope. "I'll write Granny's name and address on the front of the envelope," says Aunt Maria. "I'll draw a heart on the back," says Rosa.

"Let's look at the envelope," says Aunt Maria. "It has four sides. There are two long sides and two short sides. It is a rectangle. The stamp goes in the corner of the envelope. This stamp is a square. It has four sides and all the sides are the same length," says Aunt Maria.

"Let's put the letter in the mailbox before the mail carrier comes," says Rosa. "Does our mail carrier drive to Granny's house?" asks Rosa. "Not ours," says Aunt Maria. "Our mail carrier takes our letter to the main post office. A truck takes Granny's letter with many others to the main post office in Granny's town. Then a different mail carrier will take our letter to her," says Aunt Maria.

Rosa and her Aunt Maria take the letter to the mailbox. It is at the end of their driveway. Aunt Maria says, "Let's put the flag up so the mail carrier knows we have a letter to send."

On the way back to the house, Rosa sees her friend Eunice playing in the yard. "Come in and let's make some valentines!" Rosa says. Eunice walks over to Rosa's house.

Rosa gets scissors, pencils, crayons, and red and white paper to make valentines. "First," says Rosa, "we can cut a heart shape out of paper. A heart has curved lines and a point." "Next," says Eunice, "we write a special message on the heart and color it." "We can write a friend's name on it," says Rosa. "Last, we put the valentine in our friend's valentine box. It's like a mailbox for valentines," says Rosa.

"Let's write messages to our friends on these valentines. We'll sign our name on the back," says Eunice. Here is what some of their valentine cards say:

"To Manuel - Super Kid!, from Rosa"
"To Jose - Be My Friend, from Eunice"
"To Ann - I Love You, from Rosa"

Rosa says, "I have a very special card. It is for Aunt Maria. It says 'I Love You, from Rosa.'" "I'll make one for my Aunt, too," says Eunice. Rosa and Eunice show Aunt Maria all the valentines they have made.

"I think we need one more," says Aunt Maria. "Who for?" asks Rosa. "We need one for the puppy," says Aunt Maria. "But I can't think of the best name for the puppy," says Rosa. "Everyone needs a name. A name is important," says Aunt Maria.

Rosa looks at the puppy and says, "What should I name you?" The puppy looks at Rosa and says, "Arf! Arf!"

Valentine's Day Story - Stick Puppets

Instructions: Have child color then cut out each character. Paste each character to the end of a tongue depressor or popsicle stick.

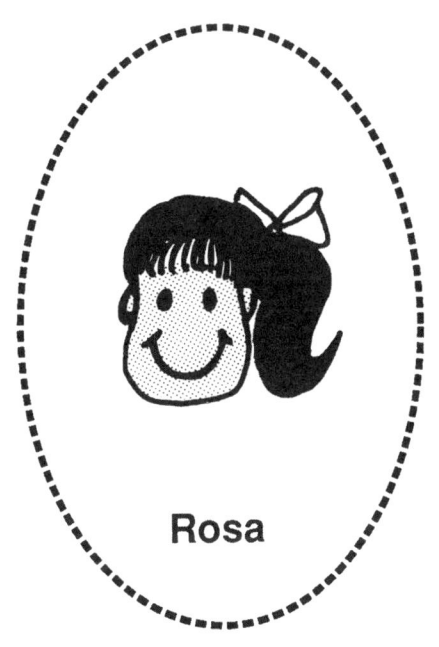

Rosa

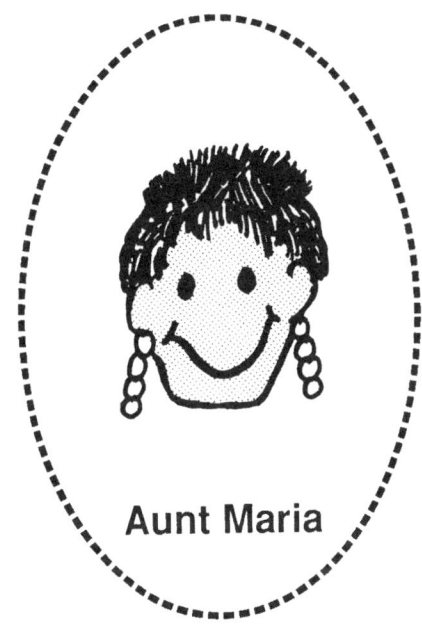

Aunt Maria

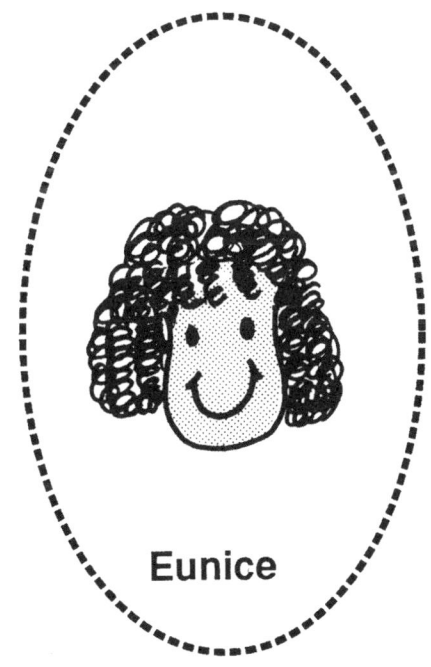

Eunice

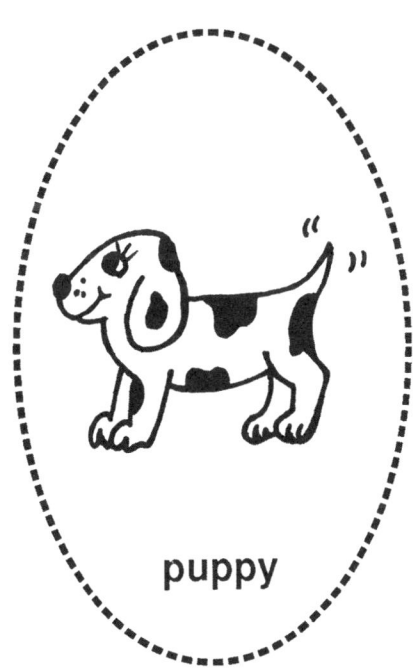

puppy

Rhyming Time

<u>**Instructor**</u>: Reproduce stick puppets (page 113). Have child color and cut out. Paste each character or figure to the end of a tongue depressor or popsicle stick.

Hopping Frog

A frog hopped by on Valentine's Day,
"Be my valentine," I heard him say.
Then he croaked and hopped real high,
So high he almost touched the sky!

My Dog

My dog likes to wag his tail,
Especially when he brings me mail.
On Valentine's Day he brings sweet wishes,
Big red hearts and candy kisses.

Be My Valentine

I love you,
Do you love me?
Please say yes
And my Valentine you'll be!

The Mail Carrier

It can be snowing,
The wind can be blowing.
The mail carrier is always here.
Let's give him a great big cheer!

Valentine's Day

Valentine's is a happy day,
We can show love in a special way.
A big red heart on a pretty card,
It really isn't very hard.

Who?

I got a pretty Valentine,
It said "I love you."
The person didn't sign it,
It just said, "Guess Who?"

<u>**Instructor**</u>: Have the child learn one poem and recite it using a stick puppet.

<u>Other Suggestions/Activities</u>

- Sentence Completion: Read a poem and leave off the last word in a line. Have the child complete the line by saying the word.

- Rewrite a poem on large chart paper. Have the child draw a picture to go with the poem. Place on bulletin board.

Rhyming Time - Stick Puppets

Valentine's Day - Worksheet 48

Instructions: Have child color then cut out each character. Paste each character to the end of a tongue depressor or popsicle stick.

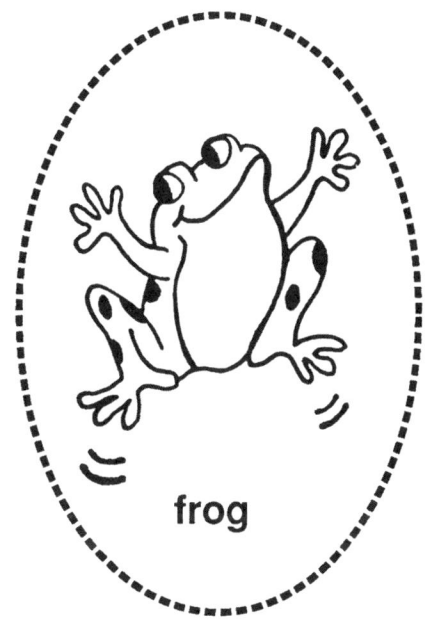

frog

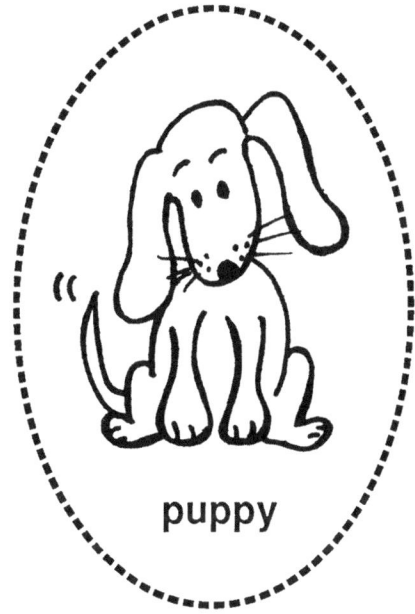

puppy

heart

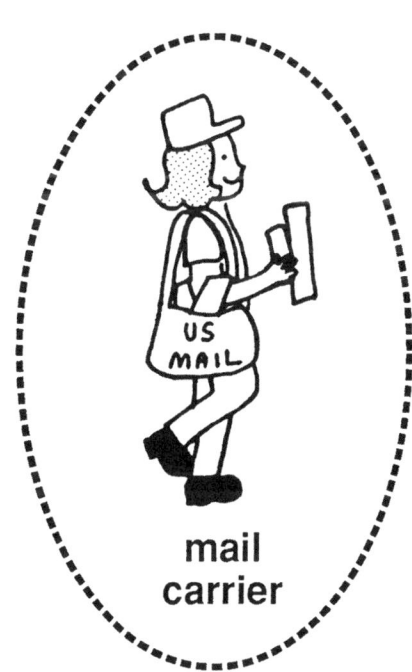

mail
carrier

113

Let's Talk About Famous Americans

Famous Americans - Worksheet 49

Introduction to Famous Americans

<u>Instructor</u>: Tell the child about George Washington, Abraham Lincoln and Martin Luther King, Jr.

Ex: We are going to learn about three famous Americans. They are George Washington, Abraham Lincoln, and Martin Luther King, Jr. We celebrate their birthdays because they worked hard to make our country free for all of us.

Concepts to Emphasize

<u>George Washington</u>: Birthday - February 22, first U.S. President, known as the Father of Our Country, had the 1st U.S. flag made, picture on a dollar bill and quarter

<u>Abraham Lincoln</u>: Birthday - February 12, 16th U.S. President, wanted all people to be free, liked to read, lived in a log cabin, wore a stove - pipe hat, picture on penny

<u>Martin Luther King, Jr</u>. - Birthday - January 18, became a minister, made speeches, wanted black and white children to go to school together, received Nobel Peace Prize

Core Vocabulary

Use the picture cards (pages 116 and 117) to introduce the Famous Americans core vocabulary. Have the child color the pictures. The pictures may be cut out and mounted on light cardboard. Describe each picture. Tell about the size, color, particular attributes of each object.

Match-up Activity

Reproduce two of each picture to make a set. Have the child find the matching pictures after you scramble them.

Other Suggestions/Activities

- After discussing how these famous Americans helped us, encourage the child to name any other people who also help us today. Ex: policemen, parents, teachers, the principal. Emphasize the concept of these people helping us to be good citizens.

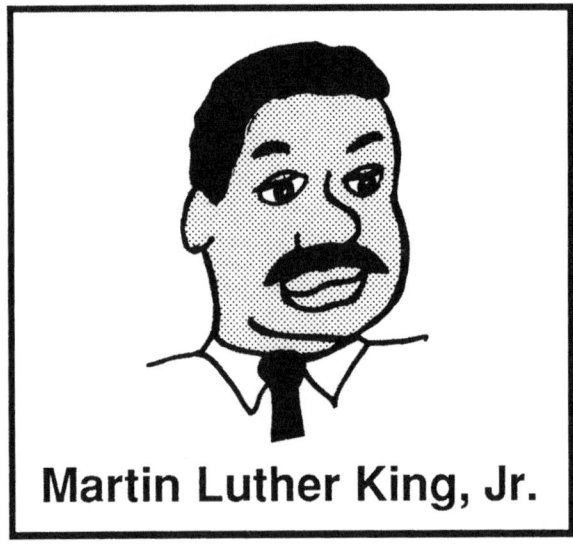

Martin Luther King, Jr.

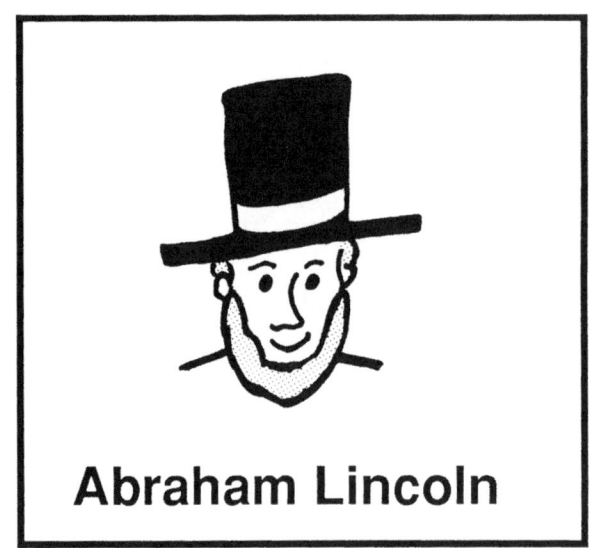

Abraham Lincoln

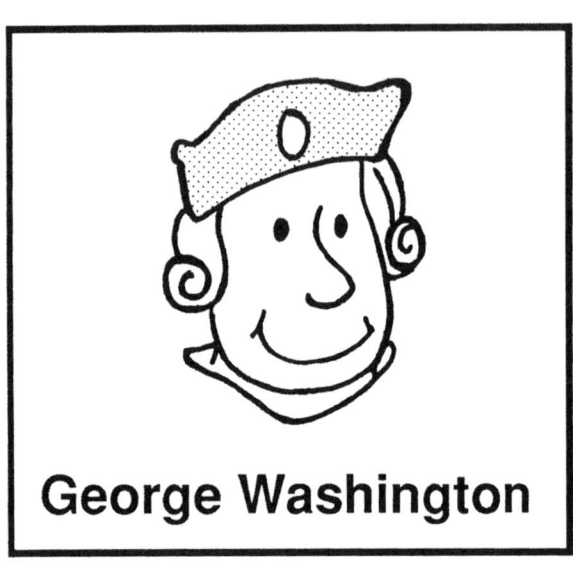

George Washington

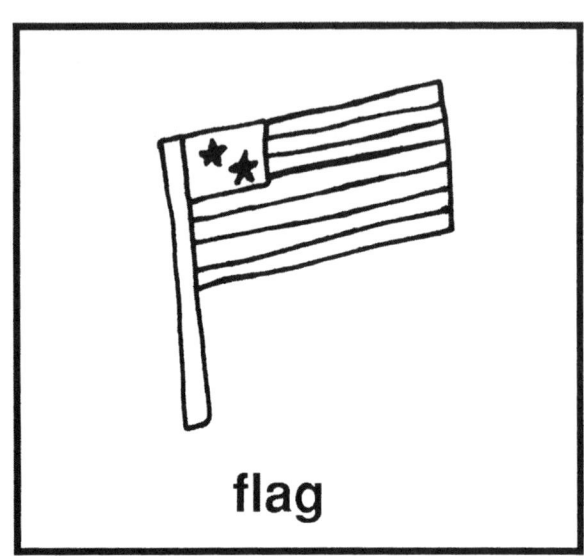

flag

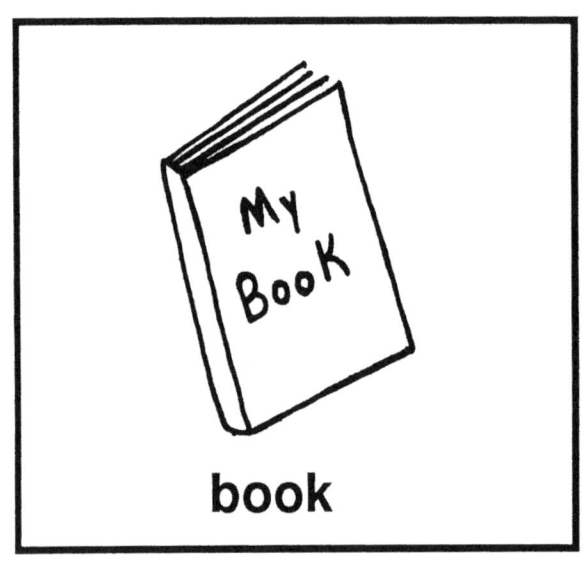

book

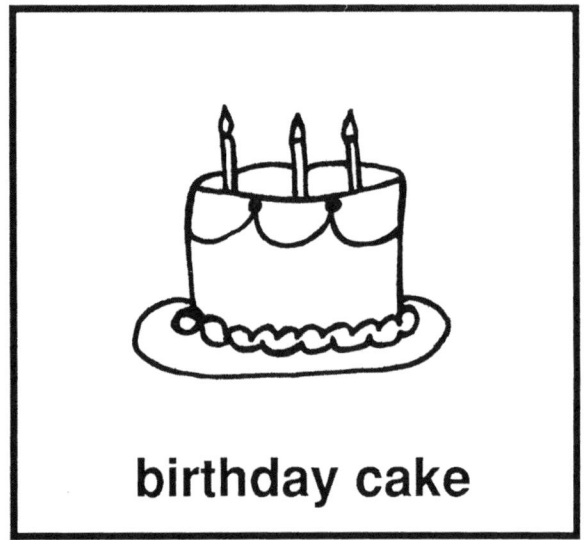

birthday cake

116

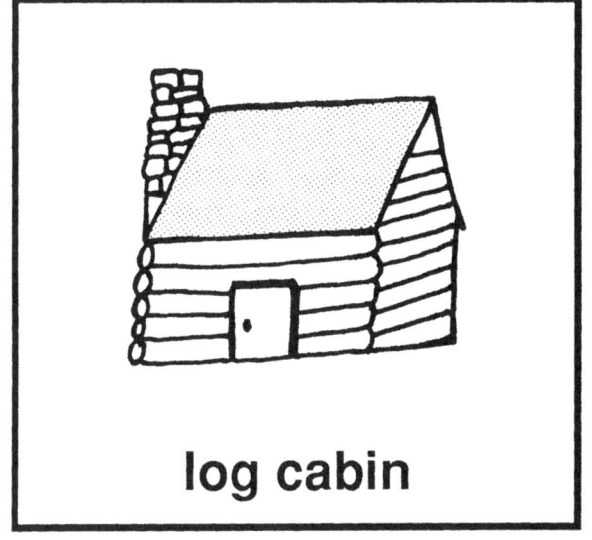

log cabin

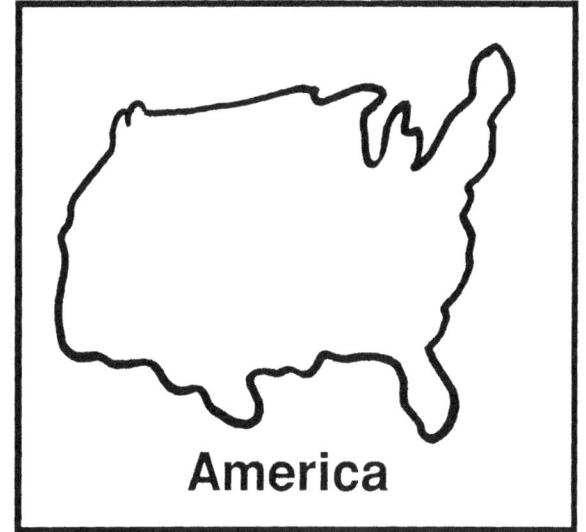

America

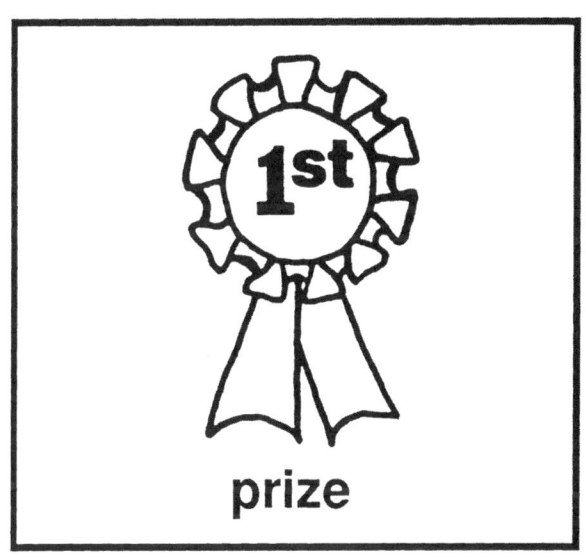

prize

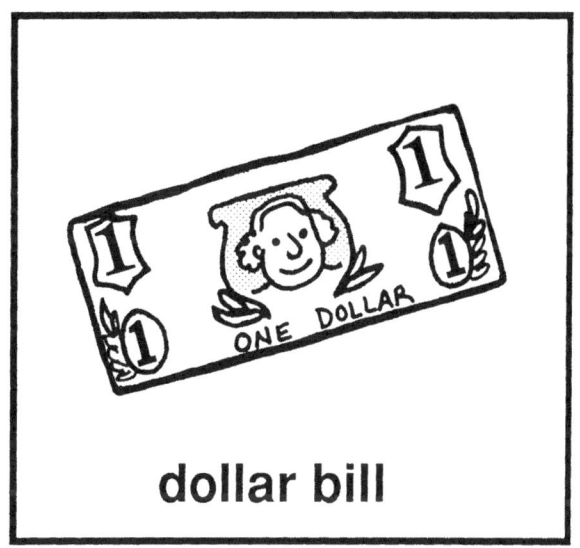

dollar bill

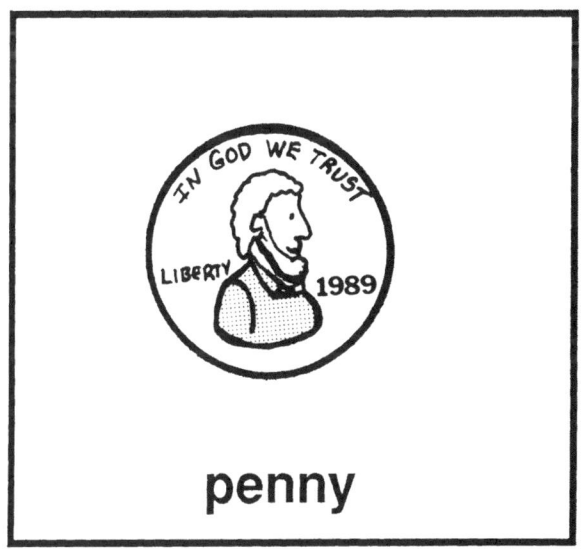

penny

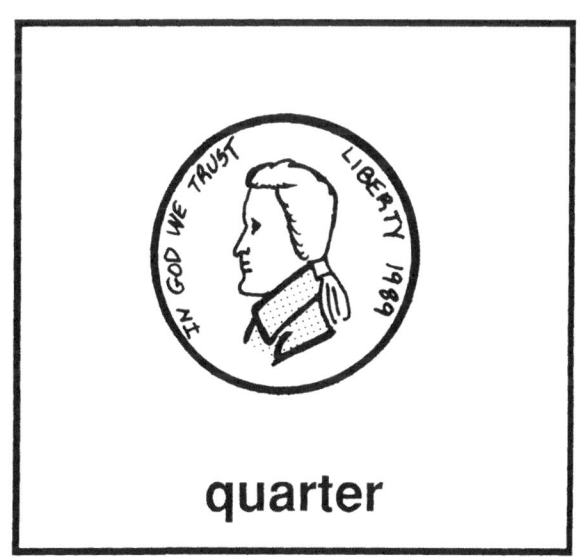

quarter

Riddle Time

Famous Americans - Worksheet 50

Instructor: Read each riddle below. Have the child choose which picture is being described. When the child chooses correctly, the picture can be colored.

1. This is a person.
   He was a minister.
   He had a dream.
   He wanted black and white
     children to go to school together.
   Who was he?
   (Martin Luther King, Jr.)

2. This is a person.
   He was tall.
   He had a beard.
   He was our 16th president.
   His picture is on a penny.
   Who was he? (Abraham Lincoln)

3. This is a person.
   He was our first president.
   He was called "The Father
     of our country."
   His picture is on a quarter and
     on a one dollar bill.
   Who was he? (George Washington)

4. It is made of cloth.
   It is red, white, and blue.
   It has 50 stars on it.
   It has 13 red and white stripes.
   What is it? (flag)

5. It is something to eat.
   It tastes sweet.
   It has icing.
   You can put candles on it.
   What is it? (birthday cake)

6. It is made of paper.
   It has pages inside.
   We read it.
   What is it? (book)

7. It is a small house.
   It is made of logs.
   Abraham Lincoln lived in one.
   What is it? (log cabin)

8. It is money.
   It is a coin.
   It is silver.
   It is worth 25 cents.
   It has George Washington's
     picture on it.
   What is it? (quarter)

9. It is money.
   It is made of paper.
   It is shaped like a rectangle.
   It has George Washington's
     picture on it.
   What is it? (one dollar bill)

10. This is very special.
    Someone may give you this.
    Maybe you will earn one in
      speech therapy or on field day.
    Martin Luther King, Jr. got one
      for working for peace.
    What is it? (prize)

11. It is a country.
    It has 50 states.
    You live in this country.
    What is it? (America)

12. It is money.
    It is a coin.
    It is brown.
    It is worth one cent.
    It has Abraham Lincoln's
      picture on it.
    What is it? (penny)

Other Suggestions/Activities

- Have the child name each picture and color it.

- Have the child choose a picture and describe it or have the child make up his own riddle.

- Say a sentence and have the child listen for a key word, i.e. "I blew out the candles on my birthday cake." When the child hears the word birthday cake, he draws a circle around the picture.

118

Riddle Time

Famous Americans - Worksheet 50

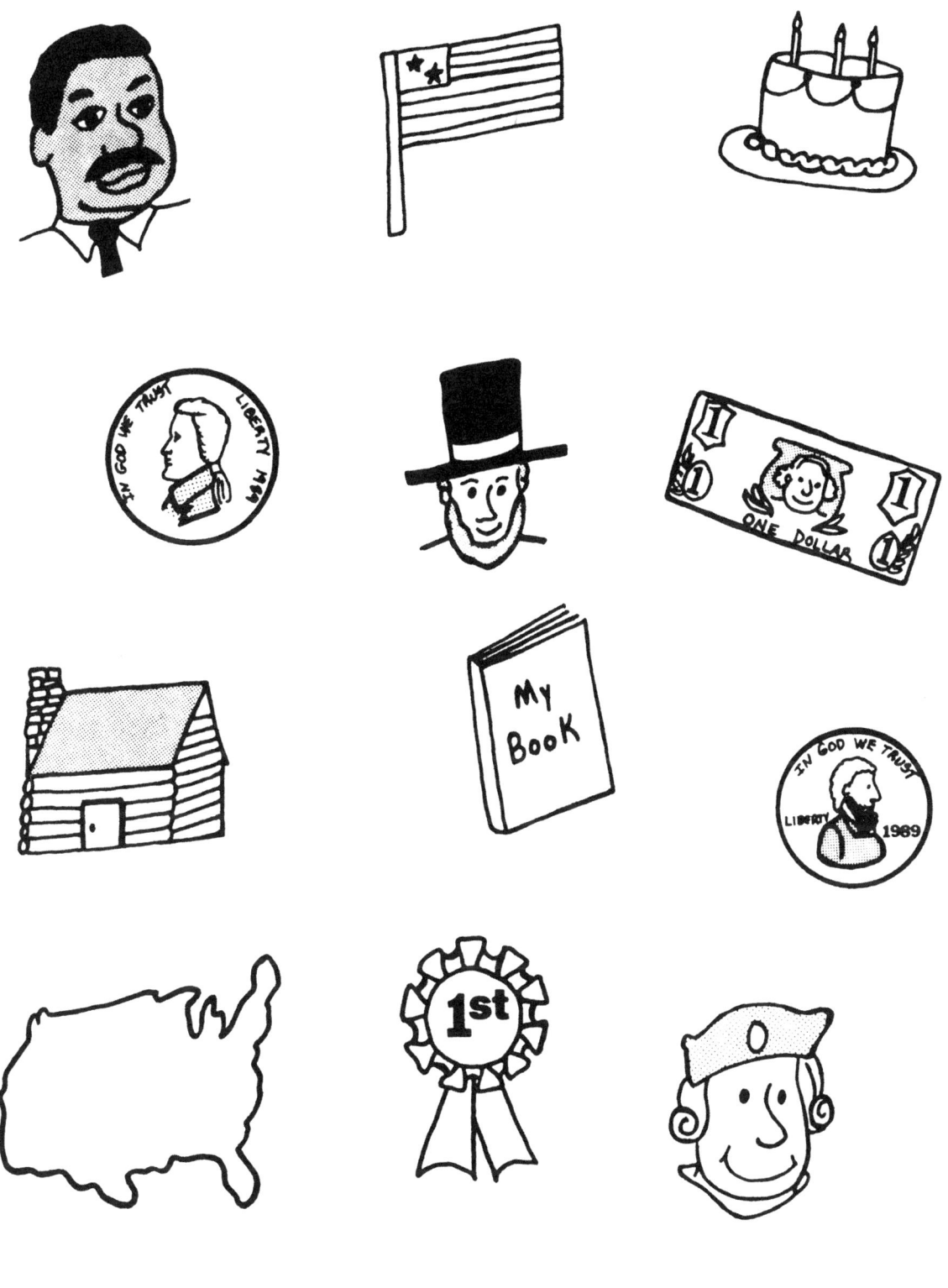

Name _____   Date _____

Lotto

Matching

Instructor: Reproduce two copies of the Lotto game for each child. Have the child color the pictures and then cut apart one set of them. The children can then match the pictures.

Lotto Game

Instructor: Reproduce two copies of the Lotto game for each child. One will be cut apart to make a "deck" of pictures. The child needs 12 markers (blocks, counters, chips, small squares of construction paper.)

The instructor says, "Listen carefully. I will pick a card and name the picture. You find the picture and put a marker on it."

Other Suggestions/Activities

- The instructor can pick a card and give a clue, description, or riddle about the picture. The child places a marker on the picture he thinks goes with the clues.

- In a group situation, the children can take turns picking a card and either naming it or giving a clue to the other children.

- Place the lotto game and deck of cards in a learning center. Color, paste on cardboard and laminate.

Lotto Game

Famous Americans - Worksheet 51

Name _____ Date _____

Five Little Pennies

Famous Americans - Worksheet 52

Instructor: Have child color and cut out pennies. Read "Five Little Pennies" poem below. As you say each verse, have child paste a penny in his bank.

Five Little Pennies

One little penny, I found in the ditch.
I put it in my bank, and now I am rich!

Two little pennies, as shiny as can be,
Maybe I'll spend them when I have three.

Three little pennies, that's one more,
I think I'll keep them until I have four.

Four little pennies, round and flat.
Maybe I should buy a brand new hat.

Five little pennies, Mom did say -
"You'd better save them for a rainy day!"

Other Suggestions/Activities

- Talk about concept of money. Use other core vocabulary words: quarter and one dollar bill.

- Have the child practice counting actual pennies.

Five Little Pennies

Famous Americans - Worksheet 52

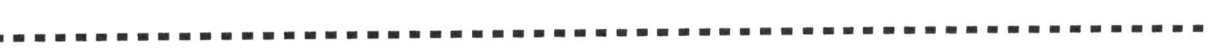

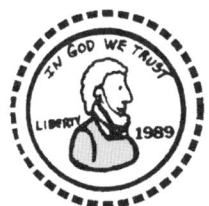 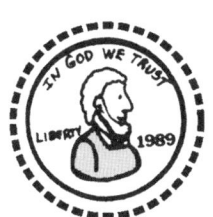 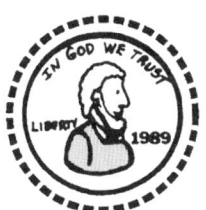 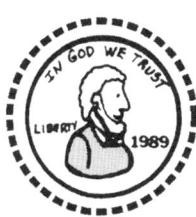 

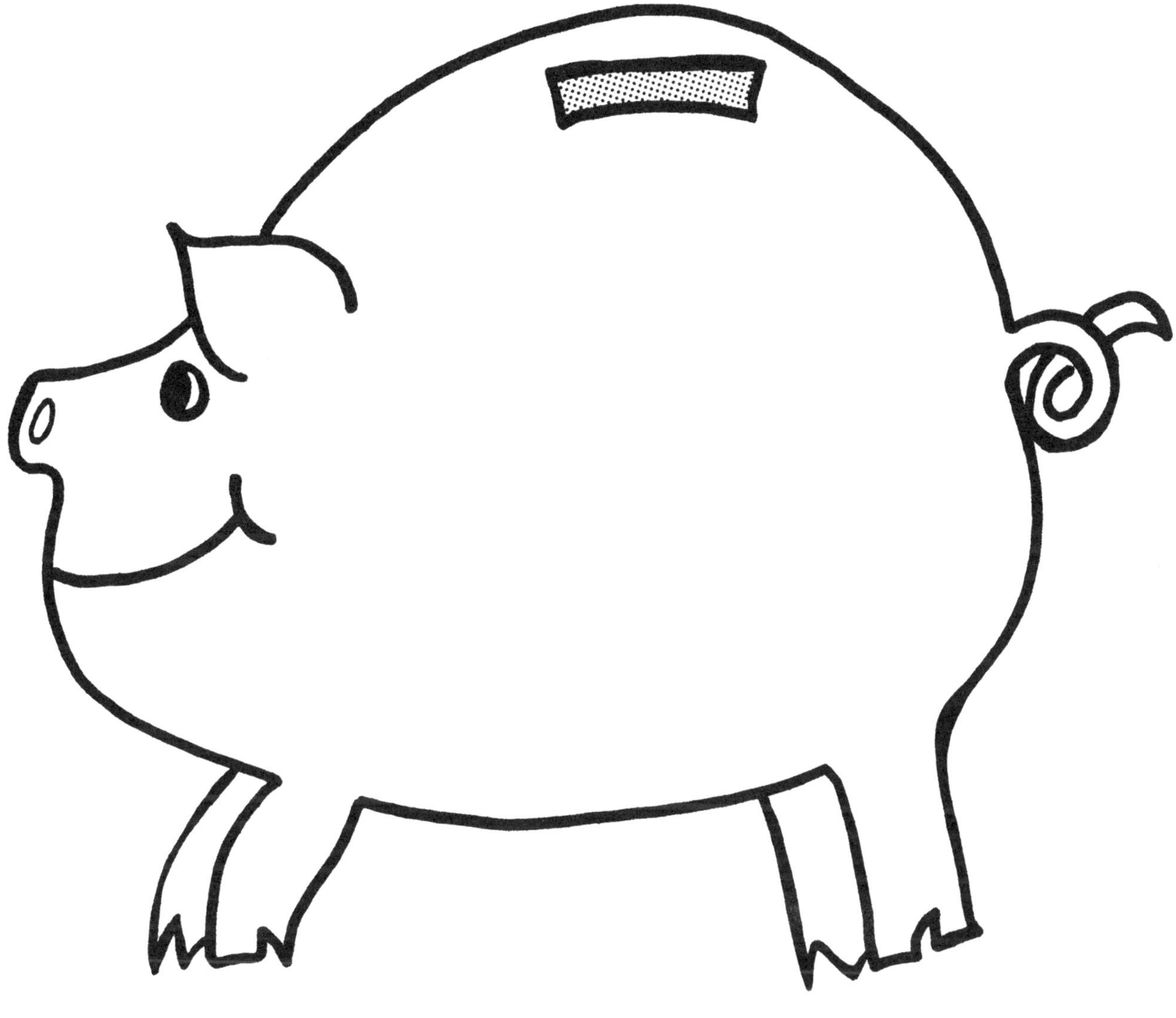

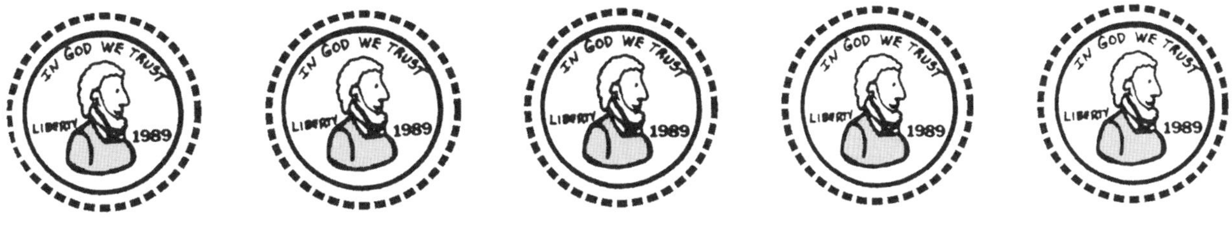

123

Flag Time

Instructor: Discuss the flag with the child. Example:

"Every country has a flag. Our country, America, has a flag that is red, white, and blue. It has 13 stripes (7 red and 6 white). It has 50 stars. There is a star for every state. The stars are white. They are on a blue rectangle. Sometimes our flag is called "Old Glory" or "Stars and Stripes." On June 14, we celebrate our flag's birthday. This is called "Flag Day."

Yes/No Questions

Instructor: "Listen carefully. I will tell you something. If I am right, answer YES. If I am wrong, answer NO." (When the child's response is correct, a part of the picture can be colored.)

1. Martin Luther King, Jr. was a minister. (yes)
2. George Washington was called Father of Our Country. (yes)
3. Abraham Lincoln was very short. (no)
4. Our flag has flowers on it. (no)
5. We read a book. (yes)
6. A birthday cake tastes sour. (no)
7. A log cabin is made of plastic. (no)
8. Martin Luther King, Jr. received a prize for peace. (yes)
9. A dollar bill has George Washington's picture on it. (yes)
10. We live in America. (yes)
11. A quarter is silver. (yes)
12. A penny is worth one cent. (yes)

Sentence Completion

Instructor: "Listen carefully. I will say a part of a sentence. When I stop, you say a word to finish the sentence." (When the child's response is correct, a part of the picture can be colored.)

1. Martin Luther King, Jr. wanted black children and white children to go to the same _____. (schools)
2. George Washington was called the Father of Our _____. (country)
3. Abraham Lincoln was our sixteenth _____. (president)
4. The flag has red and white _____. (stripes)
5. A book is made of _____. (paper)
6. We put candles on a birthday _____. (cake)
7. A log cabin is made of _____. (wood, logs)
8. When you do something special, you may earn a _____. (prize)
9. George Washington's picture is on a one dollar _____. (bill)
10. America has 50 _____. (states)
11. A quarter is worth twenty five _____. (cents)
12. A penny has a picture of _____. (Abraham Lincoln)

124

Flag Time

Name _____

Date _____

Happy Birthday

Instructor: Discuss birthdays with the child. Assist the child in learning his birthday.

How old are you?

Have the child color the birthday cake and draw candles on it to indicate how old he is.

Birthday Party

Have the child think of the kind of birthday party he would like to have and tell about it.

A Special Cake

Have the child describe his favorite kind of birthday cake and what he would like it to look like.

Other Suggestions/Activities

- Have the child tell what kind of cake he would make for one of the three famous Americans.

- Have the child say a poem (page 136) about a birthday or birthday cake.

Happy Birthday

Famous Americans - Worksheet 54

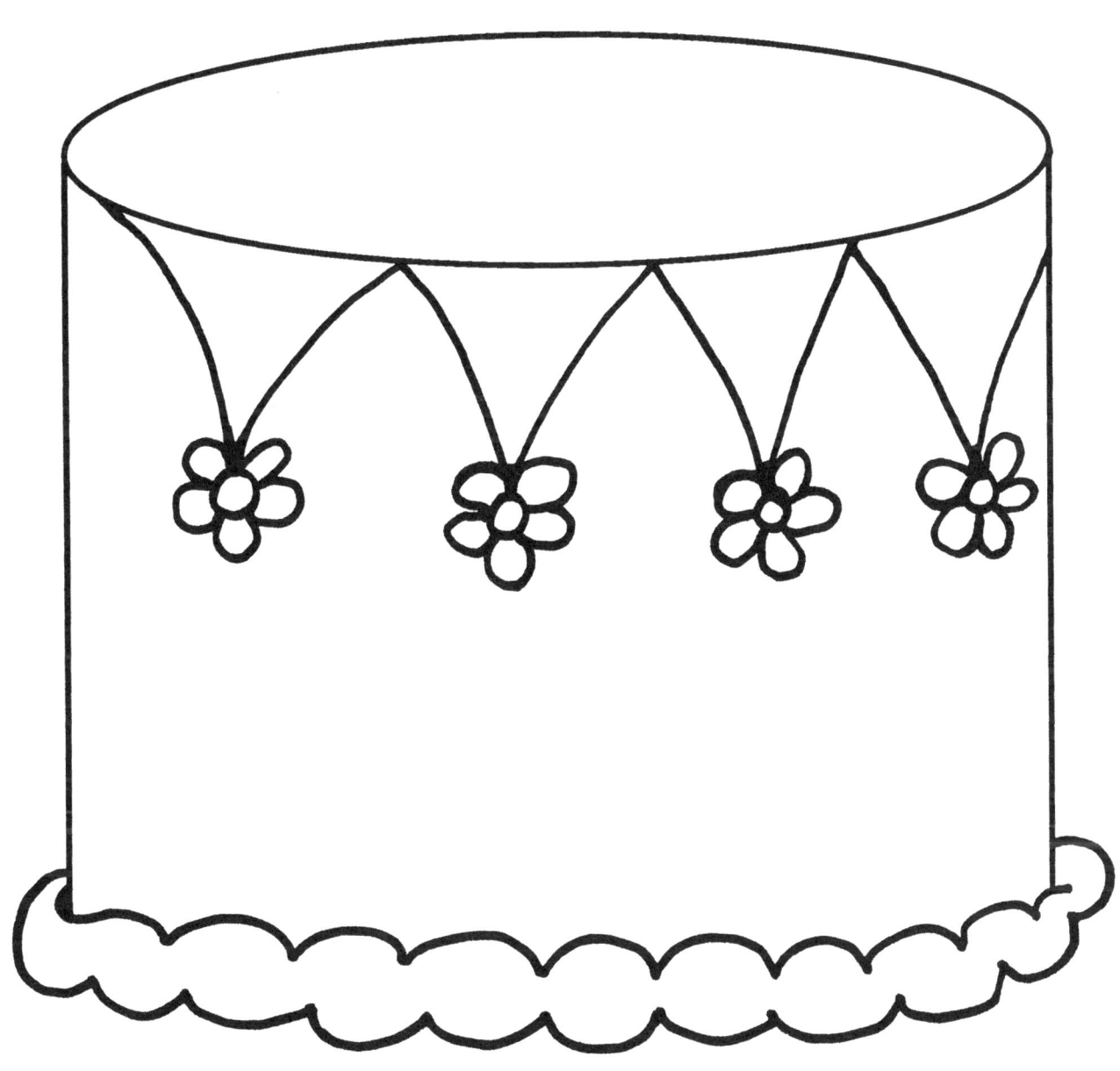

Name _____ Date _____

My Favorite Book
Famous Americans - Worksheet 55

Instructor: Discuss with the children how all of the famous Americans liked books. Read a story about Abraham Lincoln to the child.

My Favorite Book

Have the child draw a picture to represent his favorite book on the worksheet. Hang on bulletin board.

Other Suggestions/Activities

- Have the child tell about his favorite book and why it is his favorite.

- Have the child tell about one of the three famous Americans and draw a picture of him.

128

My Favorite Book

Famous Americans - Worksheet 55

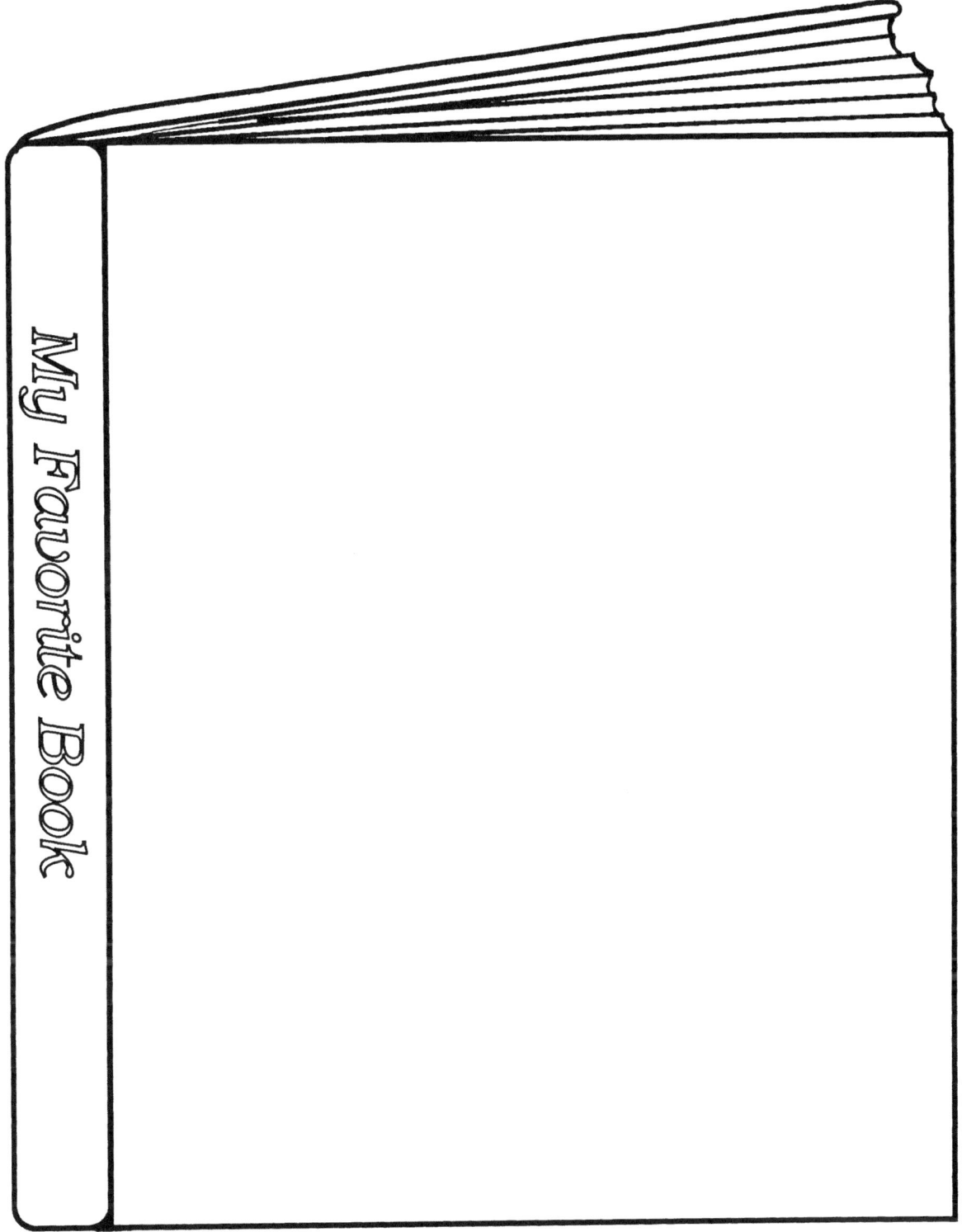

Name _____ Date _____

Prize Day
Famous Americans - Worksheet 56

Instructor: Discuss prizes with the child. Example:

"Martin Luther King, Jr. was given a special prize for peace. It was called the Nobel Peace Prize. Sometimes we get prizes. On field day, if you run very fast you may get a prize. If you do all your work in class, your teacher may give you a prize. Prizes can be many different things. They can be special ribbons, medals, money, stickers, etc. When we do something special we may get a prize."

A Prize For You

Have the student color and cut out the ribbon. Write the child's name on the prize. Think of something special about the child. Write it on the ribbon. Tell the child why he is special to you.

Ex: Johnny is a good listener.
Suzie helps clean up.

130

Prize Day

Famous Americans - Worksheet 56

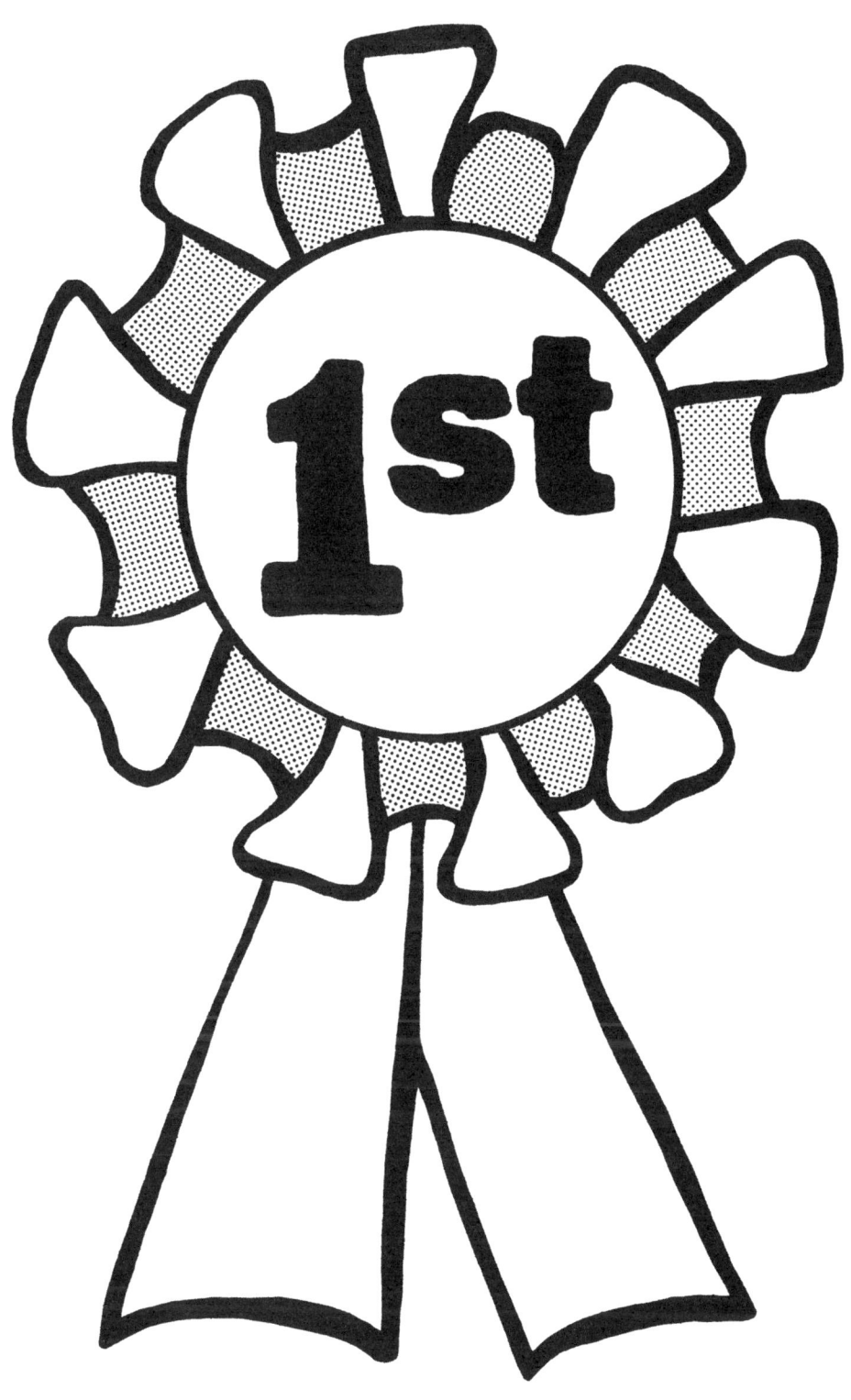

Name _____ Date _____

Famous Americans Story

Instructor: Read "Happy Birthday to All" to child. If possible, use props to assist in attending skills. (Wear a stove pipe hat like Abraham Lincoln, have small flag nearby, wear a special prize ribbon.)

Storytime

Reproduce stick puppets (page 135). Have the child color, cut out, and paste on a tongue depressor or popsicle stick. Use while telling the story or have the child hold up a stick puppet when they hear the name of their character in the story.

Use the stick puppets and have the child retell a part of the story.

Other Suggestions/Activities

- Read one paragraph at a time and ask "WH" questions.

> Ex: Paragraph 1
> Whose birthday is it?
> What are they going to have?
> How is the house decorated?

- Have the child draw a picture about the story and tell about his picture.

- Twin Day: Talk about the concept of twins. Have the child pick someone in the class and have them be "twins" for a day.

Happy Birthday to All

Characters: Eric, Darrick, Dad, Aunt Betty, Sharon, Tom

Today is a very special day! Eric and his twin brother Darrick are having their birthday party. The boys are so excited! The house is decorated with balloons and streamers.

There is a knock on the door. Aunt Betty comes in with a beautiful birthday cake. The top has chocolate icing. "Happy Birthday" is written on the cake with yellow icing. There are many other birthday party treats in Aunt Betty's shopping bag. There are birthday candles, ice cream, and a special prize for all the children.

"Wow, this is going to be a great birthday party," says Eric. "This is a special day because you are both so special," says Dad. "There are many special people with birthdays in the winter," says Aunt Betty. "Dr. Martin Luther King, Jr.'s birthday is in January." "I'd like to hear about him again," says Darrick.

"When Martin was a little boy he liked to play with his friends. They played football in the fall. They played baseball in the summer. They rode their bicycles together. One day the children said that they could not play with Martin because he was black. Martin did not understand," says Aunt Betty.

"Black children and white children did not go to the same schools. Martin thought this was not fair. Martin would dream about the day that black children and white children would go to the same school and ride the bus together. Martin loved to read books and talk to people. When he talked people would listen. Martin became a minister. He made speeches. He wanted change. He wanted his dream to come true," says Dad.

"Now, black and white children go to the same schools and ride the bus together. Many changes have been made because of Dr. King," says Aunt Betty. "Dr. King was given a very special prize. It was called a prize for peace."

Just then there is a knock on the door. Eric opens the door for his friends Sharon and Tom. "We have been talking about birthdays," says Eric. "We have too," says Sharon. "Grandmother is making a cherry pie. She has been talking about George Washington," says Tom. "He was the first president of the United States and his picture is on the quarter" says Sharon.

"There is a story that he chopped down a cherry tree," says Aunt Betty. "When his father asked him what happened, George said, 'I did it!' He always told the truth. President Washington had the first American flag made. He is known as the 'Father of Our Country.'"

"Another famous American with a winter birthday is Abraham Lincoln," says Dad. "He was the sixteenth president of the United States. When Abe was a little boy, he loved to read. He would sit up late at night in his log cabin and read. He would even have a book in his hand when he plowed the fields. One time he worked for a man three days to pay for a lost book. 'Honest Abe' they called him. When Abe grew up he had a beard and wore a stove pipe hat. He was very tall. President Lincoln wanted all people in America to be free," says Dad. "If you look on a penny, you will see Abraham Lincoln's picture on it."

The doorbell rings again. There are more children at the door. "It is time for the party to begin," says Aunt Betty. She lights the candles on the cake. The boys make a wish and blow out the candles. The children sing "Happy Birthday."

Aunt Betty gives all the children a prize. She gives a special gift to Eric and Darrick. They open their gift and inside for each one is a brand-new dollar bill with George Washington's picture on it. "Birthday parties are so much fun!" say Eric and Darrick.

134

Famous Americans Story - Stick Puppets

Instructions: Have child color then cut out each character. Paste each character to the end of a tongue depressor or popsicle stick.

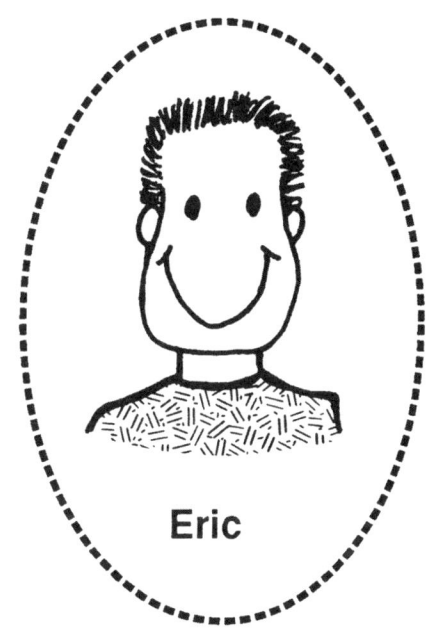

Eric

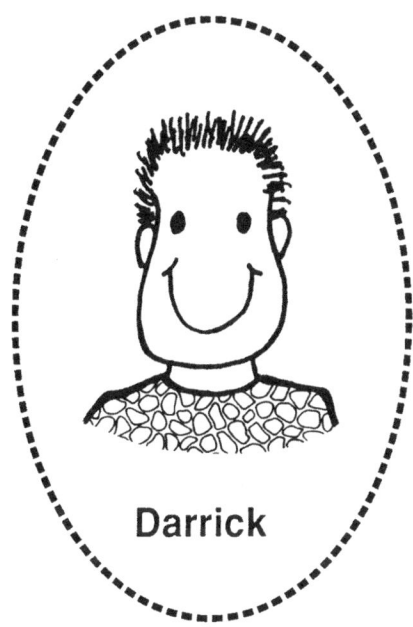

Darrick

Dad

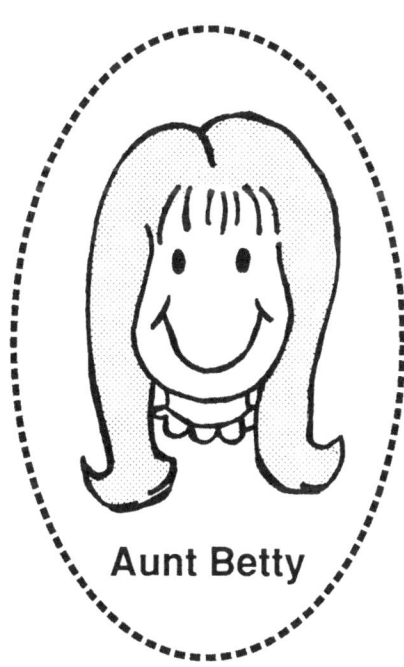

Aunt Betty

Rhyming Time
Famous Americans - Worksheet 58

<u>**Instructor**</u>: Reproduce stick puppets (page 137). Have child color and cut out.
Paste each character to the end of a tongue depressor or popsicle stick.

Poem Time

<u>**Instructor**</u>: Read a poem. Have the children hold up a stick puppet when they hear
the name of their character.

Our Flag

Red, white, and blue,
Thirteen stripes too.
A star for every state,
Our flag looks great!

Honest Abe

Honest Abe
Was very tall.
With his beard,
Hat and all!

Martin

Martin, Martin
He's our man!
He showed us how,
And now we can.

Birthday Cake

Birthday cake, I like to eat,
The chocolate ones are really neat.
Yellow icing on the top
I eat and eat - I just can't stop.

George Washington

George chopped down
The cherry tree,
He sighed and said -
"It was me!"

Happy Birthday

Blow out the candles,
Hope your wish comes true,
Cut the cake and we will sing
Happy Birthday to you!

Other Suggestions/Activities

- Sentence completion: Read a poem and leave off the last word in a line. Have
  the child complete the line by saying the word.

- Have the child learn one poem and recite it using a stick puppet.

- Rewrite a poem on large chart paper. Have the child draw a picture to go with the
  poem. Place on bulletin board.

136

Rhyming Time - Stick Puppets

Famous Americans - Worksheet 58

Instructions: Have child color then cut out each character. Paste each character to the end of a tongue depressor or popsicle stick.

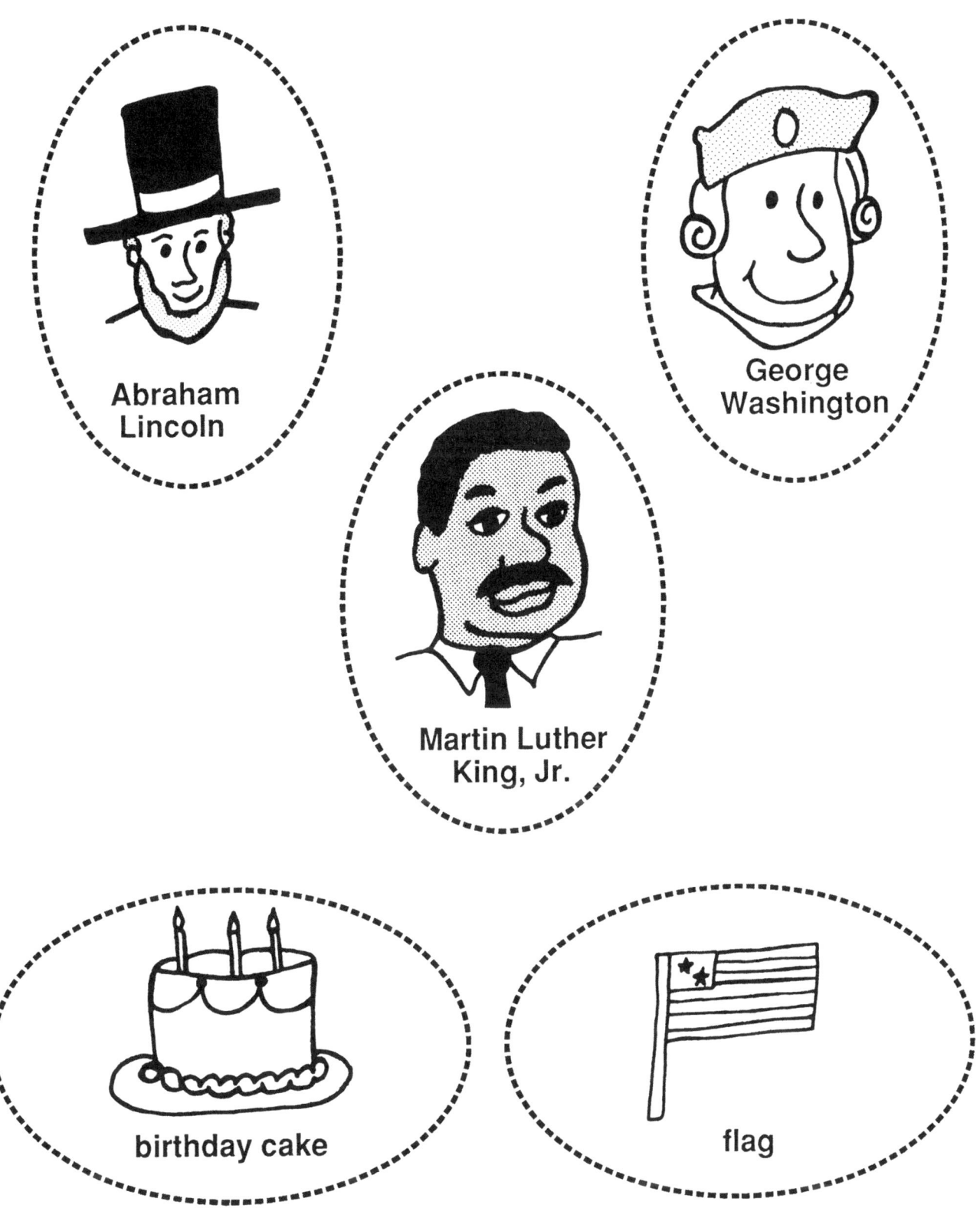

Abraham
Lincoln

George
Washington

Martin Luther
King, Jr.

birthday cake

flag

137

Let's Talk About St. Patrick's Day

Introduction to St. Patrick's Day

Instructor: Tell the child about St. Patrick's Day

Ex: St. Patrick's Day is on March 17th. This day began a long time ago in a country called Ireland. It honors a man named St. Patrick. St. Patrick was a very special person in Ireland. When Irish people came to America, they brought their traditions with them for everyone to share and appreciate. On St. Patrick's Day, people wear something green. They may wear a paper shamrock. A shamrock has three leaves and looks like clover. There are parades and parties. People like to eat corned beef and cabbage and a special stew.

When we think of St. Patrick and Ireland, we think of leprechauns. Leprechauns are tiny make-believe, elflike people. There are many legends or stories about them.
It is said that a leprechaun will reveal a buried pot of gold to anyone who catches him. There is also a legend about a pot of gold at the end of the rainbow.

St. Patrick's Day also tells us that spring is on its way. The weather begins to change. It may be windy. It is a good time for children to play outside and fly kites.

Core Vocabulary

Use the picture cards (pages 140 and 141) to introduce the St. Patrick's Day core vocabulary. Have the child color the pictures. The pictures may be cut out and mounted on light cardboard. Describe each picture. Tell about the size, color, particular attributes of each object.

Match-up Activity

Reproduce two of each picture to make a set. Have the child find the matching pictures after you scramble them.

Other Suggestions/Activities

- Reproduce the picture cards. Use in conjunction with the gameboard (page 157).

- Reproduce two of each picture. Use to play concentration game.

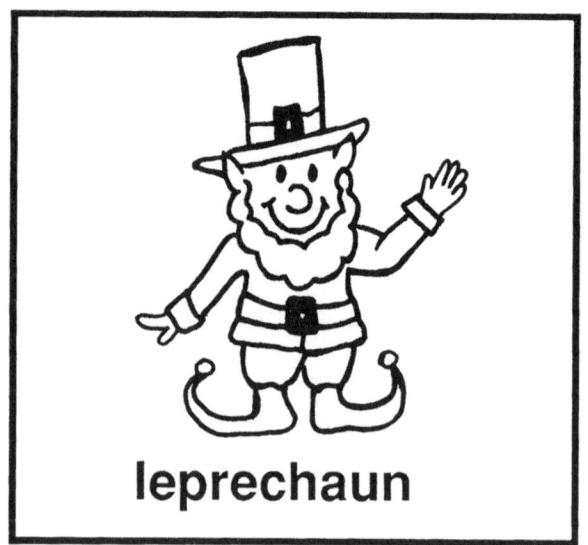

leprechaun

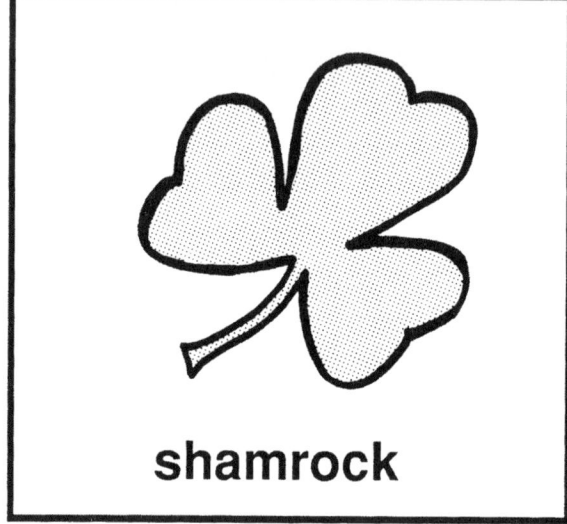

shamrock

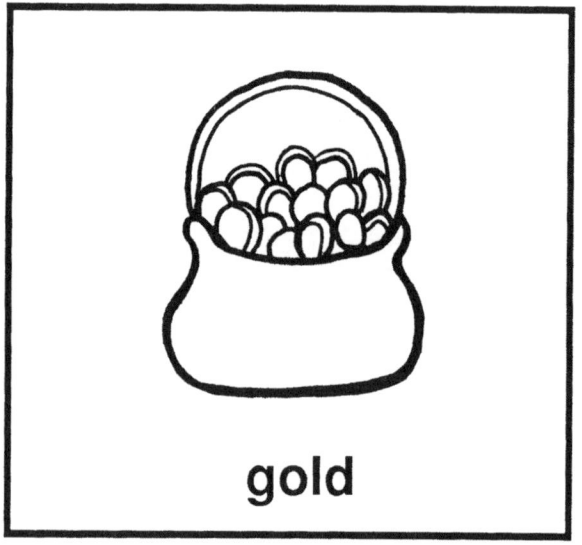

gold

140

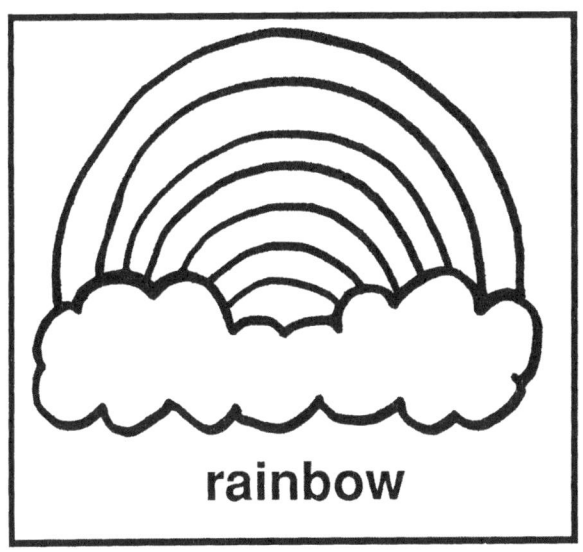

rainbow

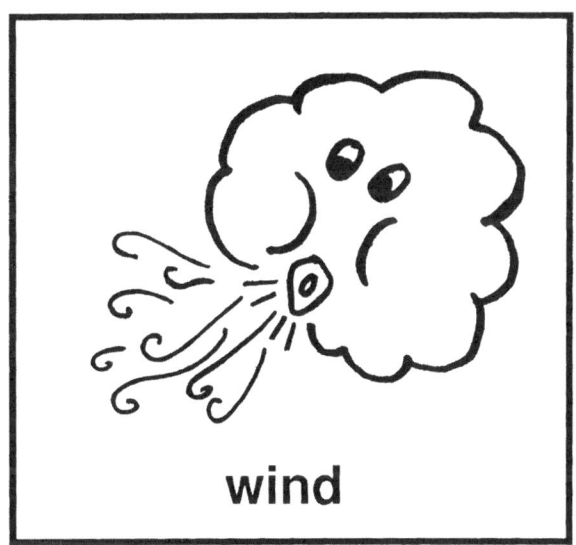

wind

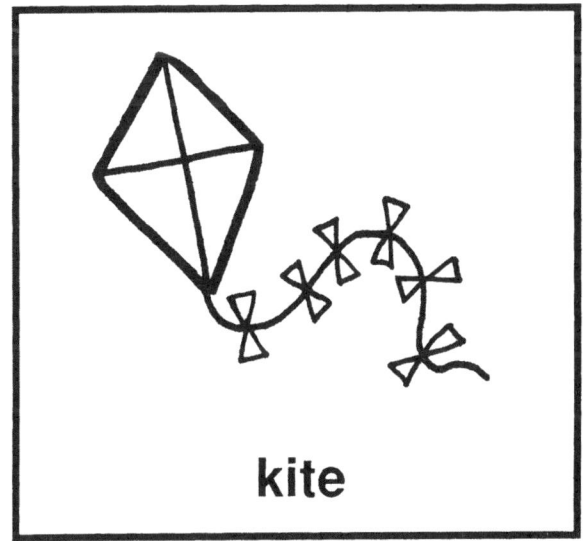

kite

Riddle Time

Instructor: Read each riddle below. Have the child choose which picture is being described. When the child chooses correctly, the picture can be colored.

1. It is green.
   It is a plant.
   It has 3 leaves.
   You may wear one on
     St. Patrick's Day.
   What is it? (shamrock)

2. It is a make-believe person.
   It is little
   It looks like an elf.
   It has a beard.
   It wears a green hat.
   Some people say it
     is invisible.
   What is it? (leprechaun)

3. It has many colors.
   You see it in the sky.
   You see it after it rains.
   What is it? (rainbow)

4. It is very shiny.
   It is bright yellow.
   In fairy tales, you can find it
     at the end of a rainbow.
   What is it? (gold)

5. It is made of paper or plastic.
   It can be different shapes
     and colors.
   Some have long tails.
   It needs wind to fly.
   Children play with it in spring.
   What is it? (kite)

6. It is part of our weather
     in spring.
   You can feel it, but
     you can't see it!
   It blows the trees.
   What is it? (wind)

Other Suggestions/Activities

- Have the child name each picture and color it.

- Have the child choose a picture and describe it or have the child make up
  his own riddle.

- Say a sentence and have the child listen for a key word, i.e. "The <u>wind</u> is
  blowing." When the child hears the word <u>wind,</u> he draws a circle around the
  picture.

Riddle Time

St. Patrick's Day - Worksheet 60

Name _____ Date _____

Find the Gold
St. Patrick's Day - Worksheet 61

Yes/No Questions

Instructor: "Listen carefully. I will tell you something. If I am right, answer YES. If I am wrong, answer NO." (When the child's response is correct, a piece of gold can be colored.)

1. A shamrock has one leaf. (no)

2. A leprechaun is a big giant. (no)

3. A rainbow has many colors. (yes)

4. Gold is blue. (no)

5. A kite is round. (no)

6. We feel wind. (yes)

Sentence Completion

Instructor: "Listen carefully. I will say a part of a sentence. When I stop, you say a word to finish the sentence." (When the child's response is correct, a piece of gold can be colored.)

1. A shamrock is a green _____. (plant)

2. A leprechaun wears a red _____. (hat)

3. We see a rainbow in the _____. (sky)

4. The color of gold is bright _____. (yellow)

5. A kite is made of _____. (paper, plastic)

6. Wind makes trees and grass _____. (move)

Other Suggestions/Activities

- Read the child a book about leprechauns.

- Have the child color the picture and place on bulletin board.

Find the Gold

St. Patrick's Day - Worksheet 61

Can you help the leprechaun find 12 pieces of gold?
Look for the ◯ shape!

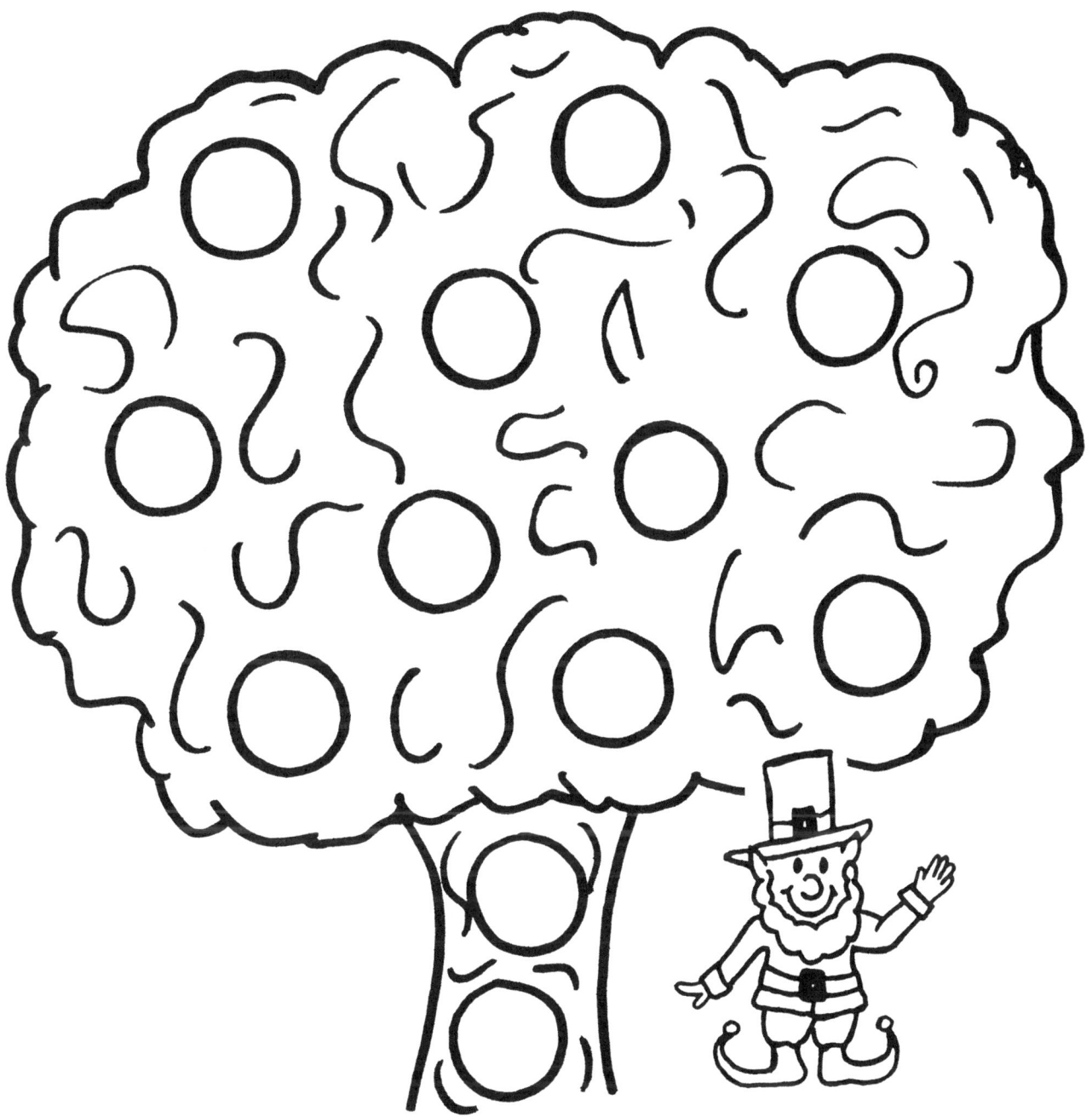

Name _____   Date _____

Over the Rainbow

St. Patrick's Day - Worksheet 62

<u>Instructor</u>: Tell the child about rainbows. Example:

> "Sometimes after it rains, you may see a rainbow. Maybe you have seen a rainbow when you play outside in the water sprinkler. When sunlight shines through drops of water it makes a rainbow. A rainbow looks like half of a circle. This shape is called an arc. The rainbow has many colors. They are red, orange, yellow, green, blue, indigo, and violet. The red is on the top edge of the rainbow."

Listen and Say

<u>Instructor</u>: This activity allows the child to listen to a question and then immediately respond. Read the statement then ask the child the question.

1. You can see a rainbow after it rains.
   When can you see a rainbow?

2. When sunlight shines through water, it makes a rainbow.
   What shines through water to make a rainbow?

3. A rainbow is shaped like an arc.
   What shape is a rainbow?

4. A rainbow is red, orange, yellow, green, blue, indigo, and violet.
   What are two colors of the rainbow?

5. The color red is on the top of the rainbow.
   What color is on the top of a rainbow?

Over the Rainbow

Reproduce the worksheet. Have the child color the rainbow.

Other Suggestions/Activities

- If possible, demonstrate how a rainbow is made by using a prism.

- Have the child learn the rainbow poem (page 154).

- Copy the rainbow poem (page 154) on large chart paper. Place on bulletin board with child's worksheet picture.

146

Over the Rainbow

St. Patrick's Day - Worksheet 62

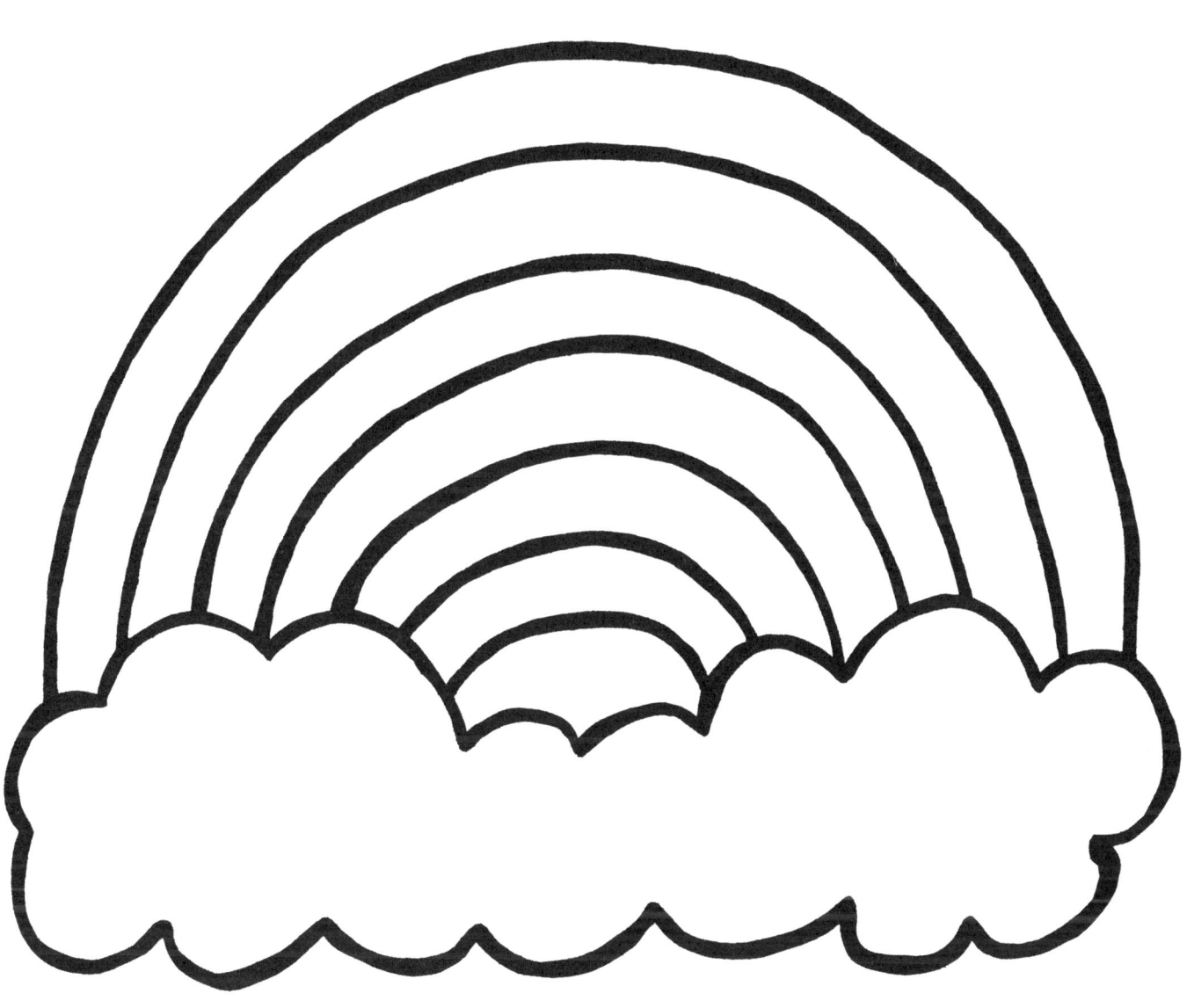

Name _____ Date _____

147

Kite Time

St. Patrick's Day - Worksheet 63

<u>Instructor</u>: Tell the child about kites. Example:

"Kites need wind to be able to fly. Kites can be many different shapes, colors, and sizes. They can be flat and shaped like a diamond. These kites need a tail made from string and cloth. This helps to balance the kite in the wind. Kites can look like boxes or they can look like dragons or birds. People have been flying kites since very long ago."

Matching Kites

Reproduce the worksheet. Discuss concepts of same and different. Have the child draw lines to the kites that are the same.

Other Suggestions/Activities

- Have the child color the kites.

- Rewrite the kite poem (page 154) on large chart paper. Place on bulletin board with the child's kite picture.

- Bring a kite to school. Have a "Kite Flying" day if there is a safe, large open space available outside.

- Have the child learn the kite poem (page 154) and recite it.

148

Kite Time

St. Patrick's Day - Worksheet 63

Draw a line between the kites that are the same.

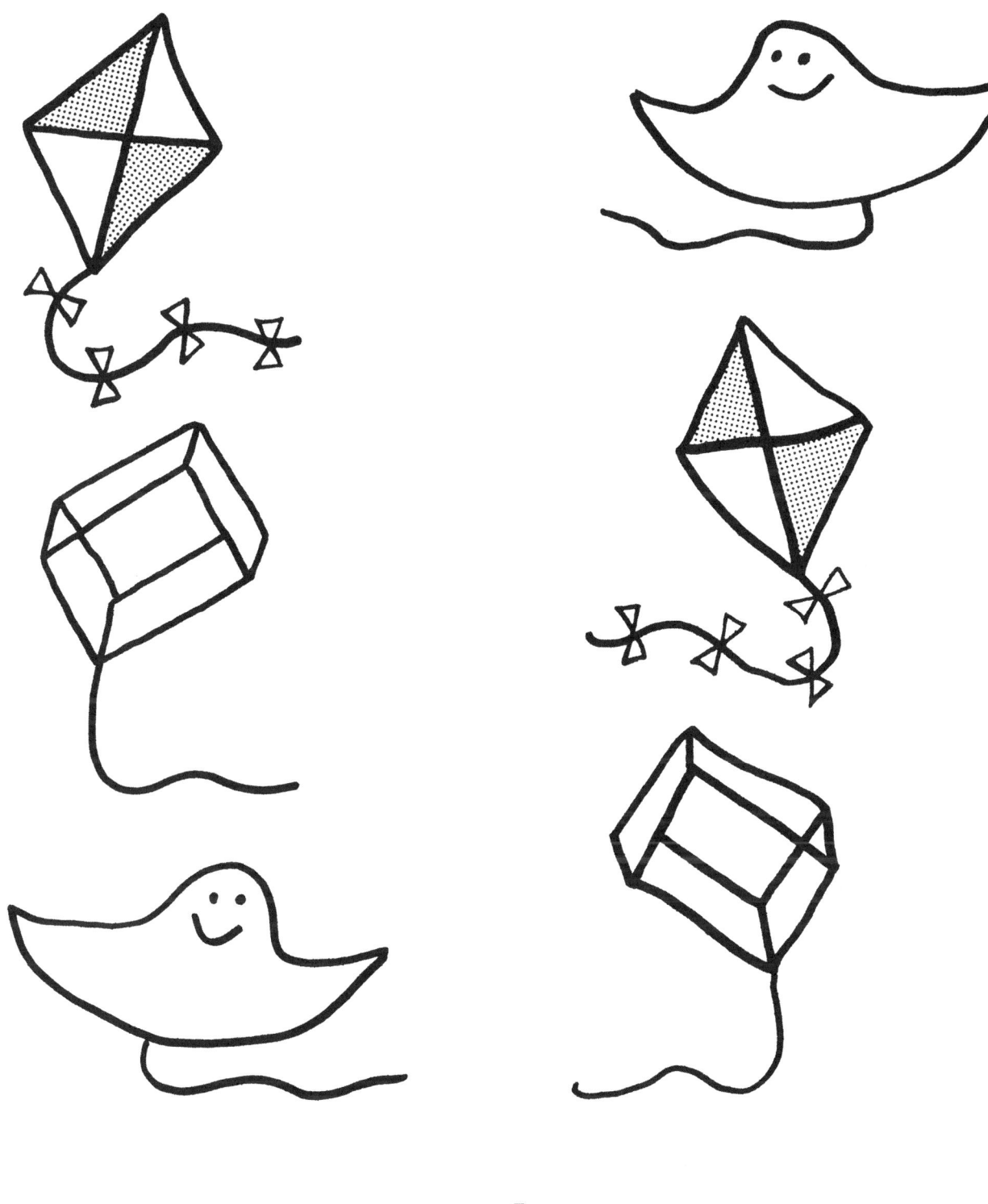

Name _____   Date _____

St. Patrick's Day Story

St. Patrick's Day - Worksheet 64

Instructor: Read "St. Patrick's Day for Grady and Shawn." If possible, use props to assist in attending skills. (Wear a shamrock, have a picture of a leprechaun, or a play pot of gold coins nearby.)

Storytime

Reproduce stick puppets (page 153). Have the child color, cut out, and paste on a tongue depressor or popsicle stick. Use while telling the story or have the children hold up a stick puppet when they hear the name of their character in the story.

Use the stick puppets and have the child retell a part of the story.

Other Suggestions/Activities

- Read one paragraph at a time and ask "WH" questions.

> Ex: Paragraph 1
> What are the boys' names?
> What is the weather like?
> Where are the boys going?

- Have the child draw a picture about the story and tell about his picture.

St. Patrick's Day for Grady and Shawn

Characters: Grady, Shawn, Grandmother

Grady's red hair is blowing in the wind. "This is a fine morning for flying kites," says Grady. "I like the weather in March." "We have big fluffy clouds and lots of wind," says Shawn. The boys are walking to their favorite kite site. It's the vacant lot at the end of the block.

"That's a nice kite," says Grady to Shawn. "It's my favorite," says Shawn. "It is shaped like a diamond. It is a flat kite, so it needs a tail for balance. I need to tie a long string to the bottom of it. Then I will take these little pieces of cloth and tie them along the string." "My kite does'nt need a tail. It is called a box kite," says Grady. "Let's get going," says Shawn.

Both boys are running and laughing. Their kites are flying high in the sky. The vacant lot is a perfect place for flying kites. It is a big open space. There are no power lines or trees. There is plenty of room to fly kites and have fun.

"March is my favorite month," says Grady. "The weather is great for flying kites." "One of my favorite days in March is St. Patrick's Day," says Shawn. "Grandma says everyone is Irish on St. Patrick's Day." "Everybody at school wears green," says Grady. "Our teacher says you better wear green or someone will pinch you."

When the boys finish flying their kites, they go to Grady's house for a snack. They smell food cooking in the kitchen. "Oh, boy! Grandma is getting ready for St. Patrick's Day. We always have corn beef and cabbage," says Grady.

The boys say hello to Grandma. She gives them a snack in the kitchen and they sit and watch her cook. Grady says, "Tell us about St. Patrick's Day, Grandma."

"On St. Patrick's Day, people wear something green. Sometimes they wear a paper shamrock. In Ireland, shamrocks grow everywhere. They look a little like our clover. They have three leaves. There are special

151

parades and parties. People visit their friends and family," says Grandma.

"There are many old legends about St. Patrick," says Grandma. "One story says that there used to be many snakes in Ireland. They say St. Patrick scared the snakes out of Ireland by beating on a drum. Another legend says that when St. Patrick's drum broke, an angel came and fixed it for him."

"There are also stories about leprechauns," says Grandma. Leprechauns are small elf-like people that live in the forests in Ireland. The stories say that leprechauns hide their gold in many different places." "Our teacher told us a story about leprechauns," says Shawn. "We pretended we were leprechauns and looked for gold sprinkled around the classroom," says Grady.

"I have heard there is a pot of gold at the end of the rainbow," says Shawn. "Have you ever seen a pot of gold at the end of the rainbow?" Grady asks his Grandmother. "No, that story is a fantasy story. It's make believe," says Grandma. The boys laugh. "Well, when I see a rainbow," says Grady, "it means I can play outside again!"

St. Patrick's Day - Stick Puppets

St. Patrick's Day - Worksheet 64

Instructions: Have child color then cut out each character. Paste each character to the end of a tongue depressor or popsicle stick.

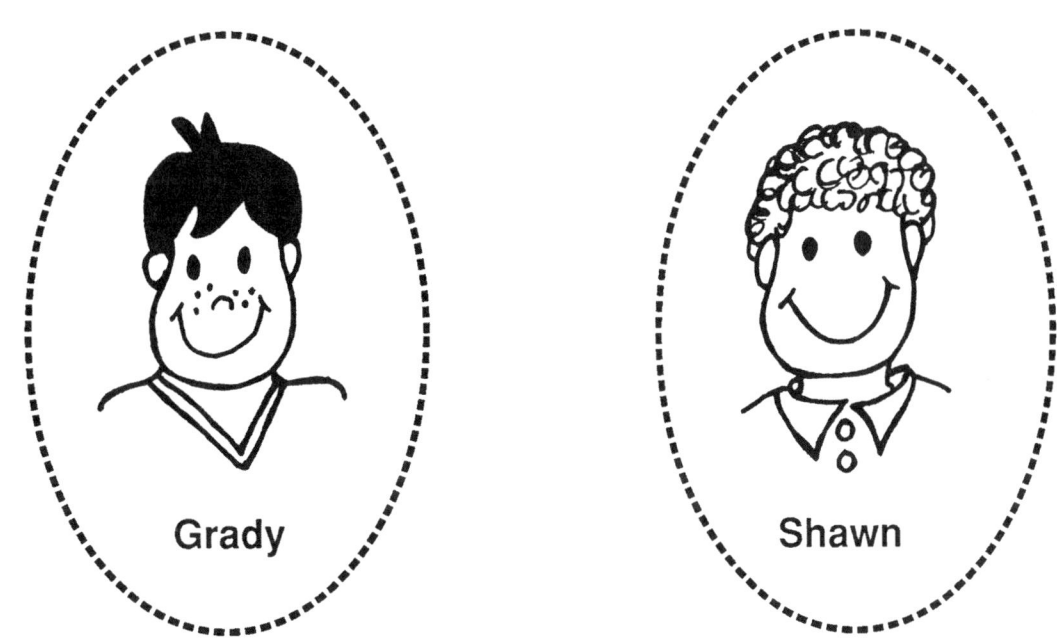

Grady   Shawn

Grandma

Rhyming Time
St. Patrick's Day - Worksheet 65

<u>Instructor</u>: Reproduce stick puppets (page 155). Have child color and cut out. Paste each character or figure to the end of a tongue depressor or a popsicle stick.

Kite

My kite flys
Into the sky.
A good, strong wind,
Will take it high!

Wearing Green

You better wear green,
On March seventeen,
Or it's a cinch,
You'll feel a pinch.

Leprechauns

Leprechauns look like little elves,
Who hide their pots of gold.
They are very hard to catch,
So I have been told.

Rainbow

A rainbow shining in the sky,
Means we can tell the rain good-bye.
Red, orange, yellow, and green,
It's the prettiest I've ever seen.

Shamrock

The shamrock is like a pretty clover,
It has three leaves and is green all over.
We wear it on St. Patrick's Day,
And hope good luck will come our way.

<u>Instructor</u>: Have the child learn one poem and recite it using a stick puppet.

Other Suggestions/Activities

- Sentence Completion: Read a poem and leave off the last word in the line. Have the child complete the line by saying the word.

- Rewrite a poem on large chart paper. Have the child draw a picture to go with the poem. Place on bulletin board.

Rhyming Time - Stick Puppets

St. Patrick's Day - Worksheet 65

Instructions: Have child color then cut out each character. Paste each character to the end of a tongue depressor or popsicle stick.

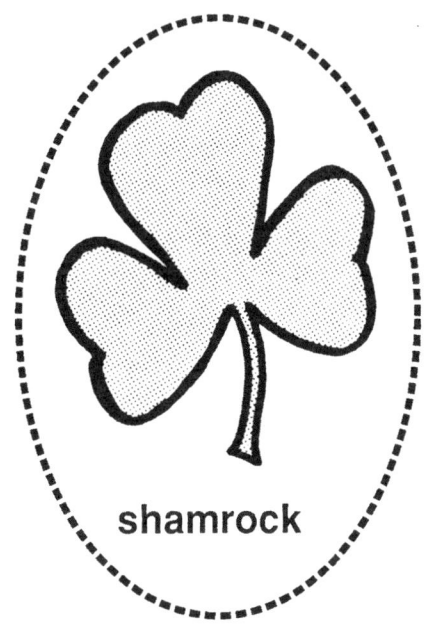

shamrock

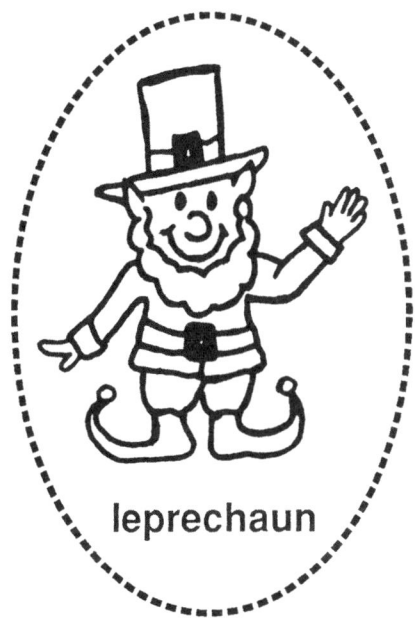

leprechaun

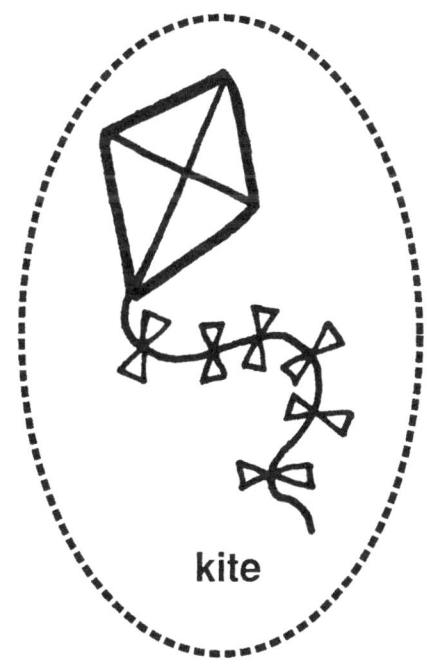

kite

rainbow

155

Lucky Leprechaun Game

Instructor: Each child selects a marker, i.e. button or pawn. Flipping a penny can be used to determine movement. Ex: Heads - move ahead one space, Tails - move ahead two spaces.

Game Time

Reproduce one set of picture cards (pages 140-141). Have the child name the picture or tell one thing about the picture before he moves.

Other Suggestions/Activities

- Use in conjunction with riddles (page 142), yes/no questions (page 144), or sentence completion (page 144).

- Use the gameboard for the development of other vocabulary, i,e, colors, numbers, basic concept words.

Lucky Leprechaun Game

St. Patrick's Day - Worksheet 66

Follow the shamrocks and help the leprechaun get to the pot of gold.

157

Let's Talk About Easter

Easter - Worksheet 67

Introduction to Easter

<u>Instructor</u>: Tell the child about Easter.

Ex: Easter is a holiday that comes in the spring. At Easter we can dye eggs different colors. We can have Easter egg hunts outside. The Easter bunny leaves us candy and treats in our Easter basket. Spring is that time of year when the weather begins to change. It gets warmer and the rain helps to make the grass and flowers grow. Baby animals are sometimes born in the spring. Birds build nests to hold their eggs.

Core Vocabulary

Use the picture cards (pages 160 and 161) to introduce the Easter core vocabulary. Have the child color the pictures. The pictures may be cut out and mounted on light cardboard. Describe each picture. Tell about the size, color, particular attributes of each object.

Match-up Activity

Reproduce two of each picture to make a set. Have the child find the matching pictures after you scramble them.

Memory Game

Place two to four cards on the table. Have the child look at the cards for a few seconds. Cover or turn over. Have the child name the pictures from memory.

Other Suggestions/Activities

- Reproduce two of each picture. Use to play concentration game.

- Play the "What would you do if?" game. Instructor chooses a picture card and asks the child a question, i.e. "What would you do if a rabbit hopped into your house?" or "What would you do if a turtle got in your soup?" Encourage the child to verbalize his feelings.

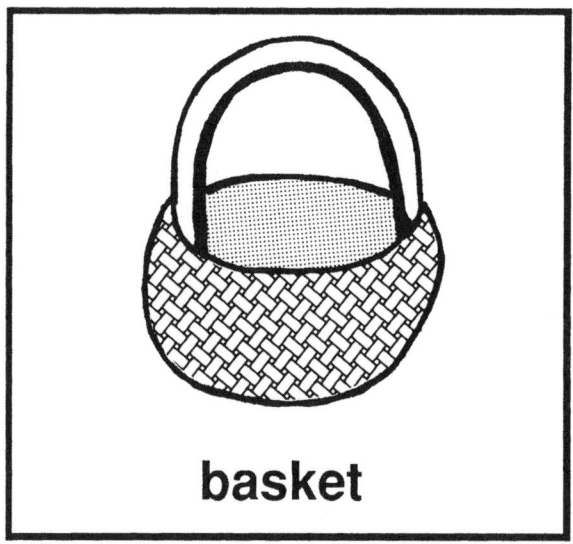

basket

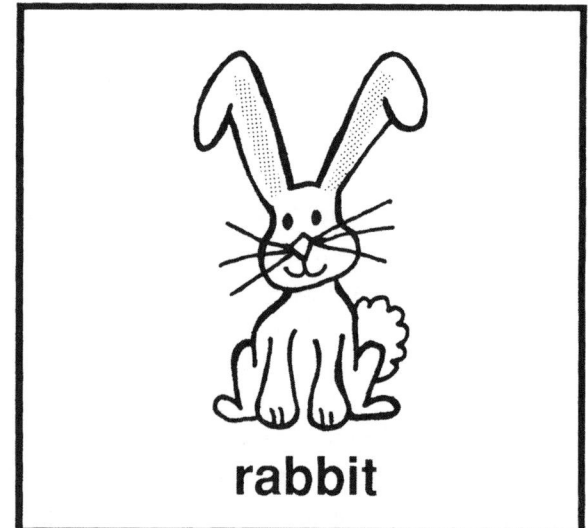

rabbit

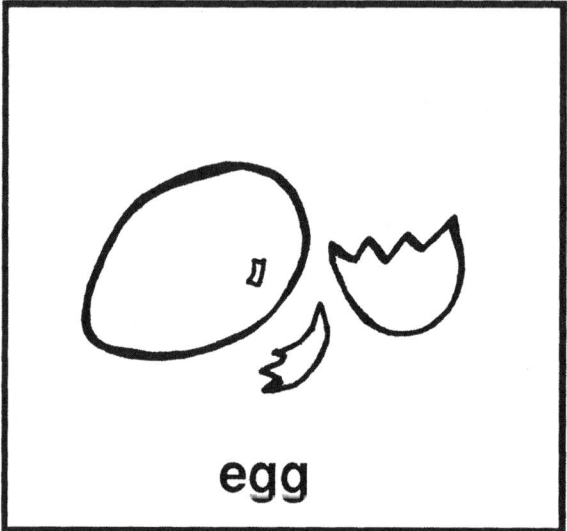

egg

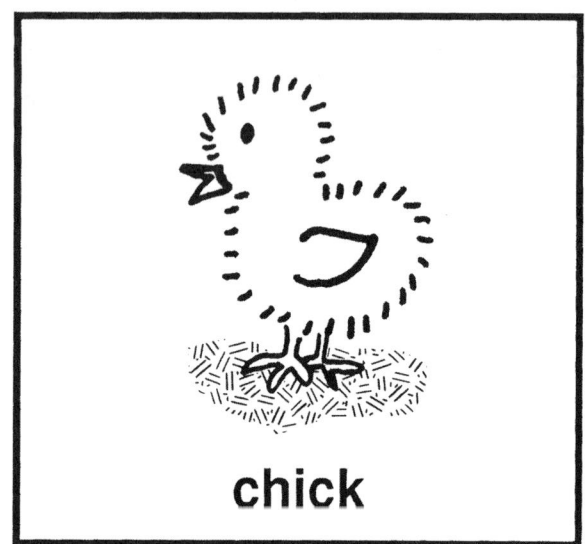

chick

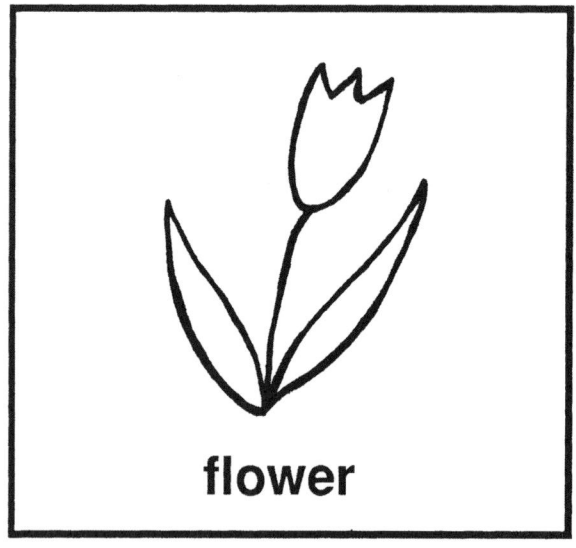

flower

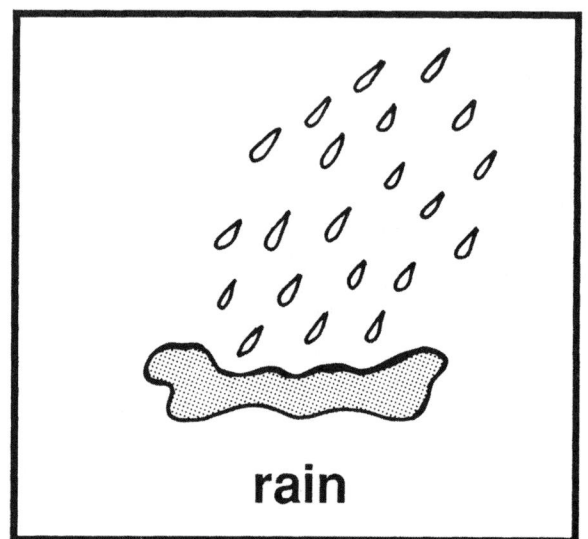

rain

160

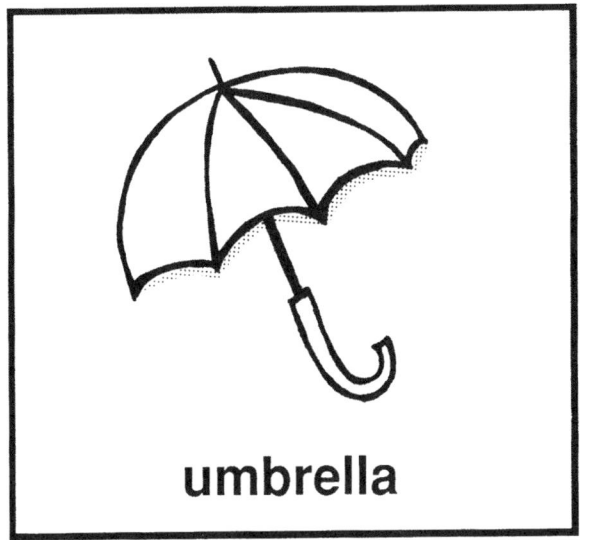

umbrella

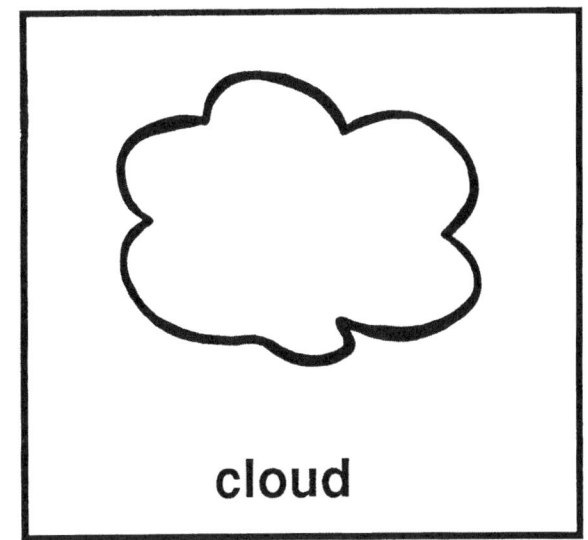

cloud

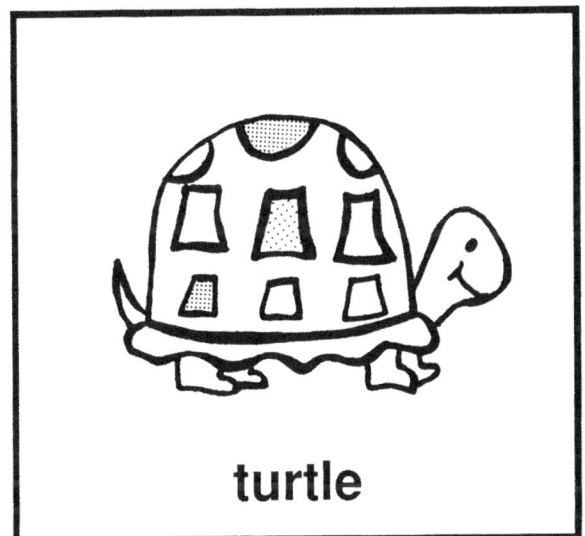

turtle

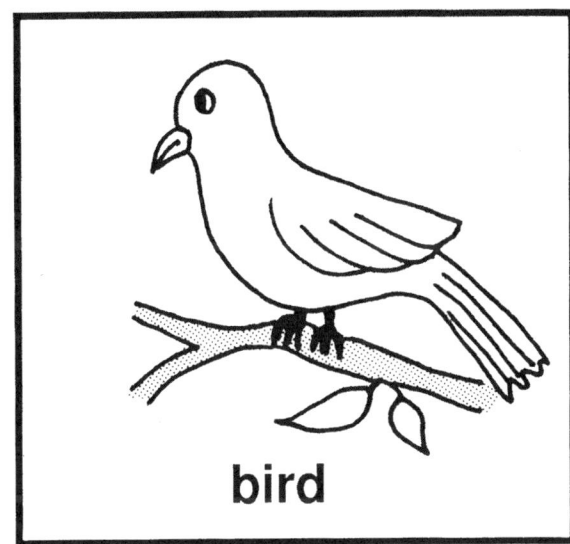

bird

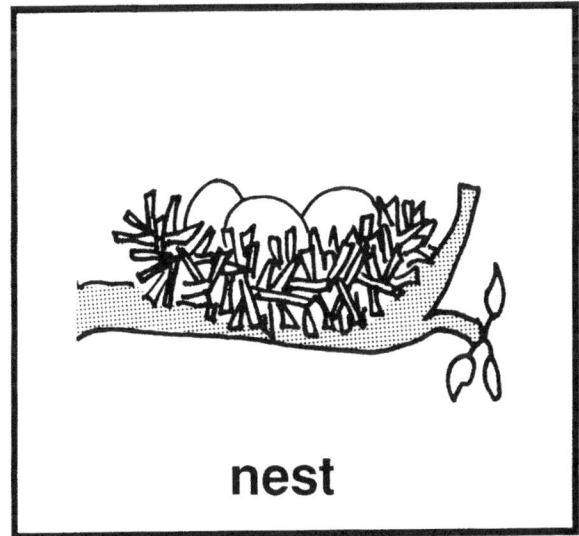

nest

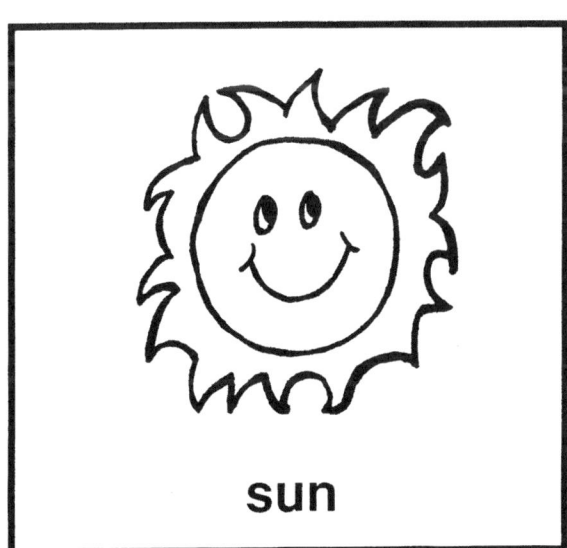

sun

Riddle Time

Easter - Worksheet 68

Instructor: Read each riddle below. Have the child choose which picture is being described. When the child chooses correctly, the picture can be colored.

1. It is made of wood or plastic.
   It has a handle.
   It has grass in it.
   We put Easter eggs in it.
   What is it? (basket)

2. It is white.
   It comes from a chicken.
   You can dye it pretty colors.
   You can eat it.
   What is it? (egg)

3. It is a baby animal.
   It hops.
   It has floppy ears.
   It can be brown or white.
   It wiggles its nose.
   What is it? (rabbit)

4. It is a baby animal.
   It is very little.
   It is very soft.
   It goes, "cheep, cheep."
   What is it? (chick)

5. It is a plant.
   It grows in spring.
   It has leaves, petals, and
   a stem.
   It smells good.
   What is it? (flower)

6. It falls from a cloud.
   It is wet.
   It is made of water.
   What is it? (rain)

7. It is hot.
   It is bright.
   You can see it in the sky.
   What is it? (sun)

8. It is an animal.
   It moves slowly.
   It has a shell.
   It can hide its body in
   the shell.
   It can be green or brown.
   What is it? (turtle)

9. It is an animal.
   It flies.
   It has feathers.
   It eats worms.
   What is it? (bird)

10. It is built by a bird.
    It holds eggs.
    It is made of twigs and grass.
    You can find it in a tree.
    What is it? (nest)

11. It floats in the sky.
    It is white.
    It is fluffy.
    Rain comes from it.
    What is it? (cloud)

12. We use this when it rains.
    We hold it over our head.
    It keeps us dry.
    What is it? (umbrella)

Other Suggestions/Activities

- Have the child name each picture and color it.

- Have the child choose a picture and describe it or have the child make up his own riddle.

- Say a sentence and have the child listen for a key word, i.e. "The turtle has a hard shell." When the child hears the word turtle, he draws a circle around the picture.

Riddle Time

Easter - Worksheet 68

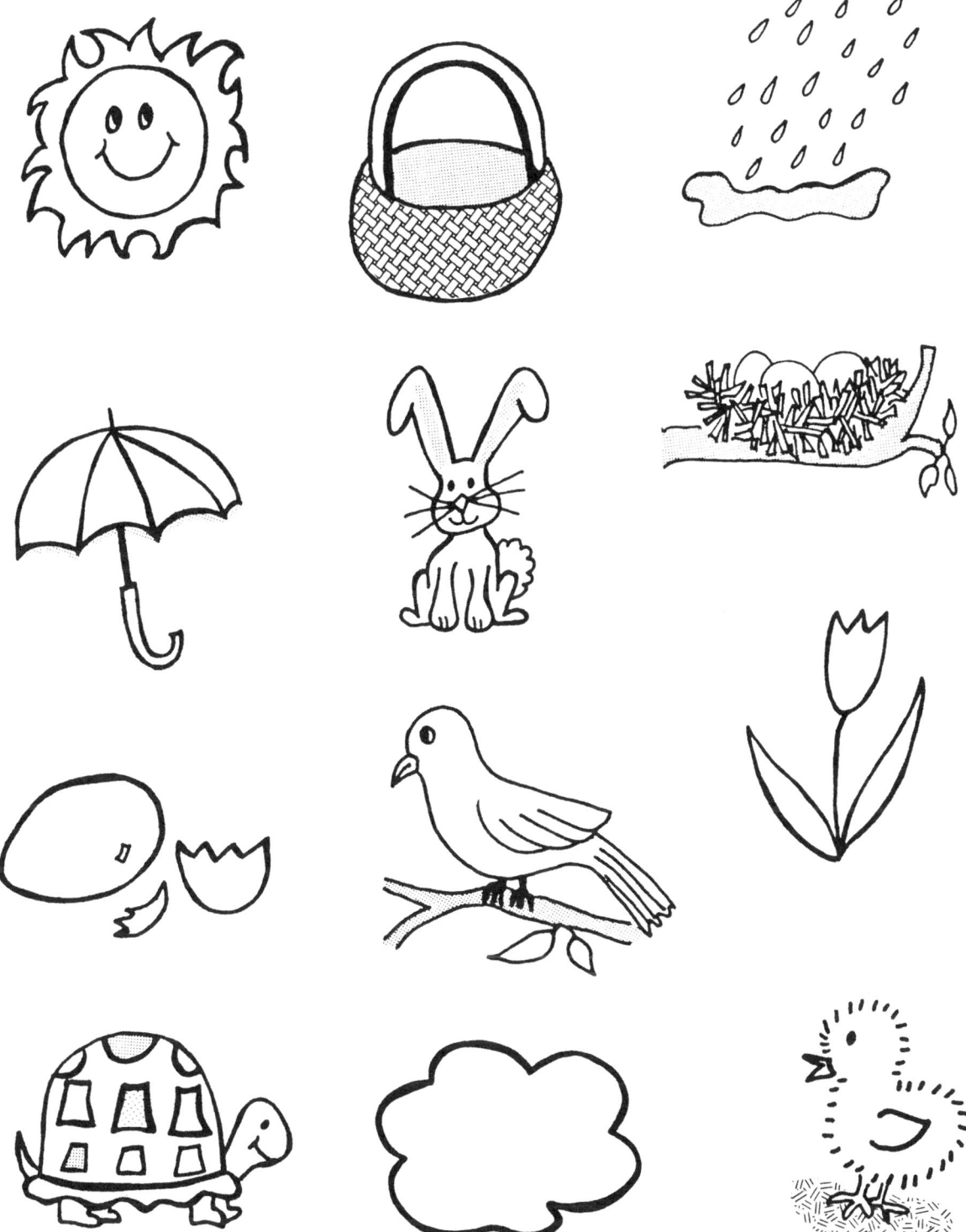

Name _____ Date _____

163

Easter Basket

Easter - Worksheet 69

Yes/No Questions

Instructor: "Listen carefully. I will tell you something. If a I am right, answer YES. If I am wrong, answer NO." (When the child's response is correct, an egg can be colored.)

1. We put rocks in an Easter basket. (no)
2. You can eat an egg. (yes)
3. Chicks say meow. (no)
4. A rabbit hops. (yes)
5. A flower is a plant. (yes)
6. Rain is made of candy. (no)
7. The sun is bright. (yes)
8. Turtles run fast. (no)
9. A bird lives in a fish tank. (no)
10. The bird nest is in the tree. (yes)
11. Clouds are white and fluffy. (yes)
12. An umbrella keeps us dry. (yes)

Sentence Completion

Instructor: "Listen carefully. I will say a part of a sentence. When I stop, you say a word to finish the sentence." (When the child's response is correct, an egg can be colored.)

1. We hold the Easter basket by its _____. (handle)
2. We dye Easter _____. (eggs)
3. A flower grows in _____. (spring)
4. A chick says _____. (cheep)
5. A rabbit has floppy _____. (ears)
6. Rain is made of _____. (water)
7. The sun is in the _____. (sky)
8. The turtle hides in its _____. (shell)
9. The bird eats _____. (worms)
10. A nest is built by _____. (birds)
11. Rain comes from _____. (clouds, sky)
12. We hold an umbrella over our _____. (head)

Easter Basket

Easter - Worksheet 69

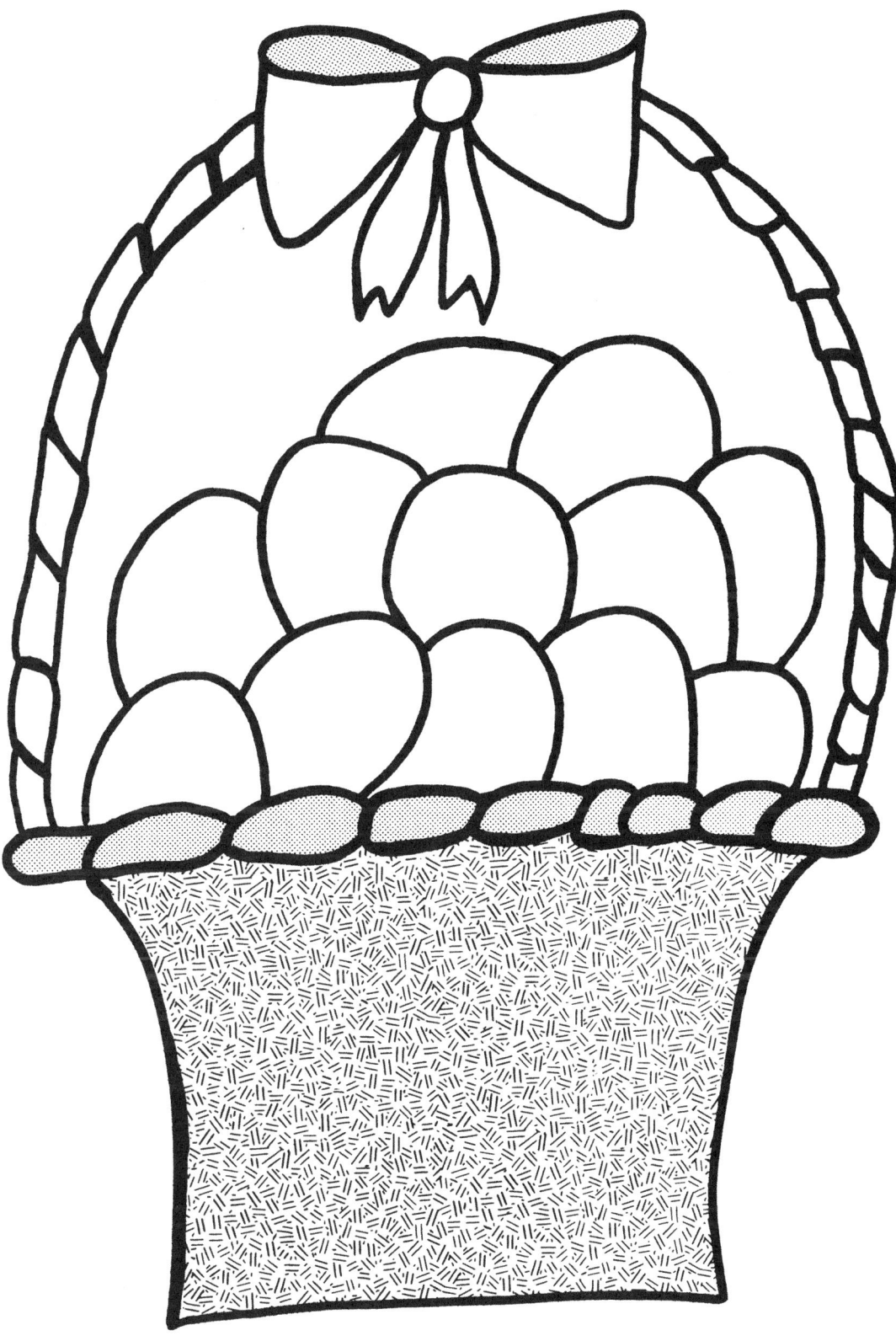

Name _____ Date _____

Following Directions

Visual Discrimination - Motor Activity

Instructor: Have the child examine each picture individually. Have the child tell you what is missing. If the child needs help getting started, try the following:

Ex: "A rabbit has big ears. Look carefully at this rabbit. Is anything missing?"

After the child tells you what is missing from each picture have him draw the missing items on the pictures.

Auditory Discrimination

Instructor: "Listen carefully and do as I say."

"Draw two ears on the rabbit."

"Draw a handle for the umbrella."

"Draw two legs on the bird."

"Draw a handle for the basket."

"Draw a head for the turtle."

"Draw a stem for the flower."

Other Suggestions/Activities

- Use for the development of basic concept words, i.e. "Draw a line over the rabbit. Draw a line under the basket."

- Use for "I am Thinking" game. The instructor says, "I am thinking of a plant. It has petals, leaves, and a stem. It smells good. What is it?"

166

Following Directions

Easter - Worksheet 70

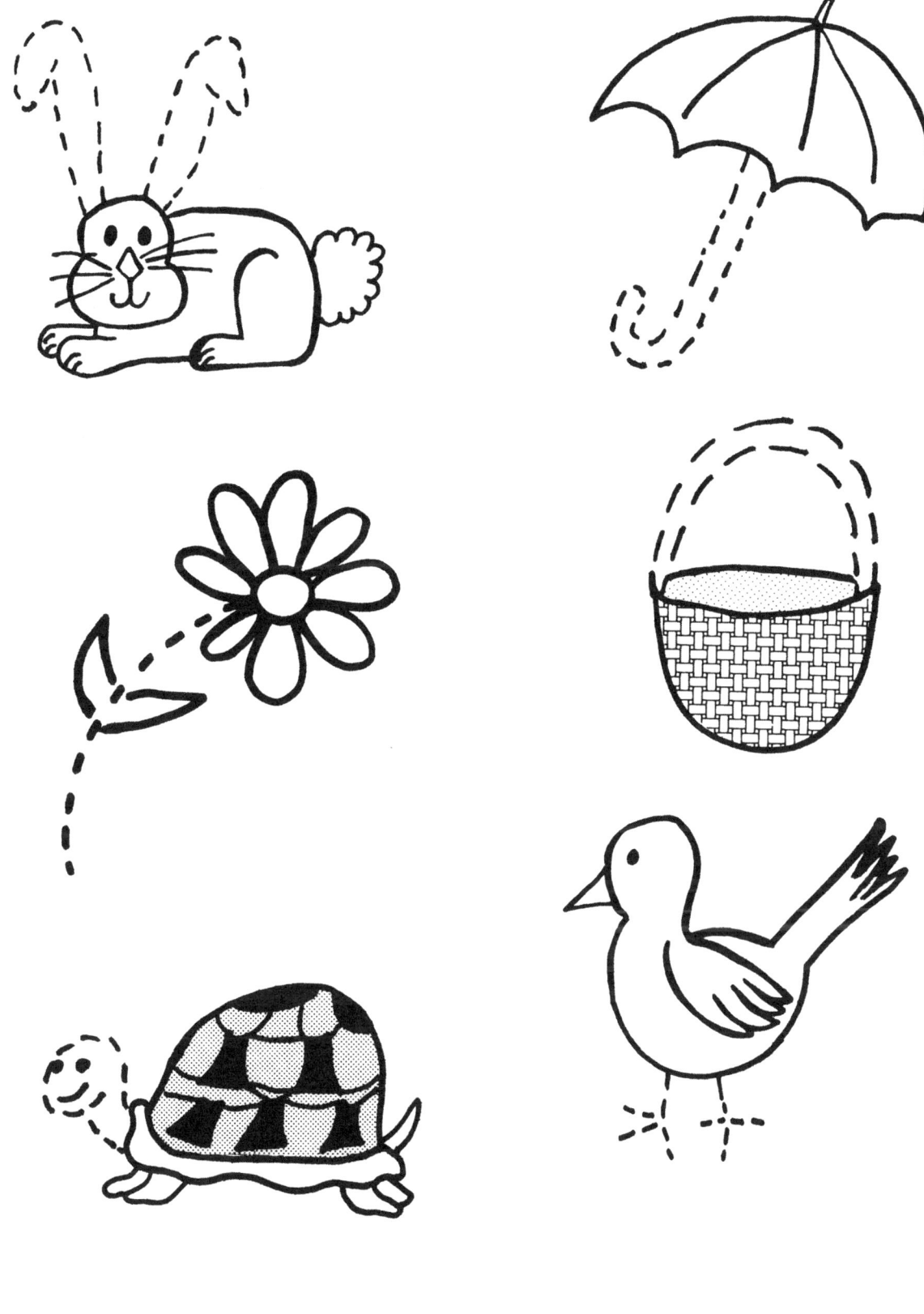

Name _____ Date _____

Five Little Chicks

Easter - Worksheet 71

Instructor: Have the child color and cut out baby chicks. Read "Five Little Chicks" poem below. As you say each verse, have child paste a chick on the page.

Five Little Chicks

One little chick, tapping on his shell,
Out he pops, looking very well.

Two little chicks, pecking on the ground,
They look so cute; bright yellow and round.

Three little chicks going "cheep, cheep, cheep."
They're not like rabbits who don't make a peep.

Four little chicks, having lots of fun,
Waiting, waiting, for the last one.

Five little chicks, right by their mother,
Four little sisters and one little brother.

Other Suggestions/Activities

- As child can repeat each verse of the poem, a chick can be pasted on the page.

- Number the chicks 1-5. Have the child practice counting.

- Make stick puppets out of the chicks on page 169. Have each child hold up a chick puppet as a verse is said.

Five Little Chicks

Easter - Worksheet 71

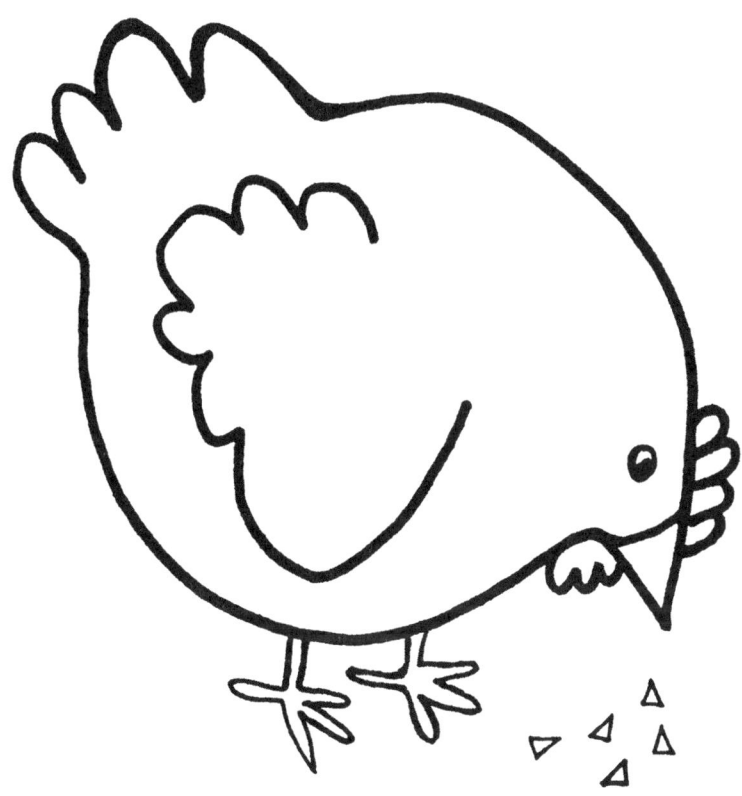

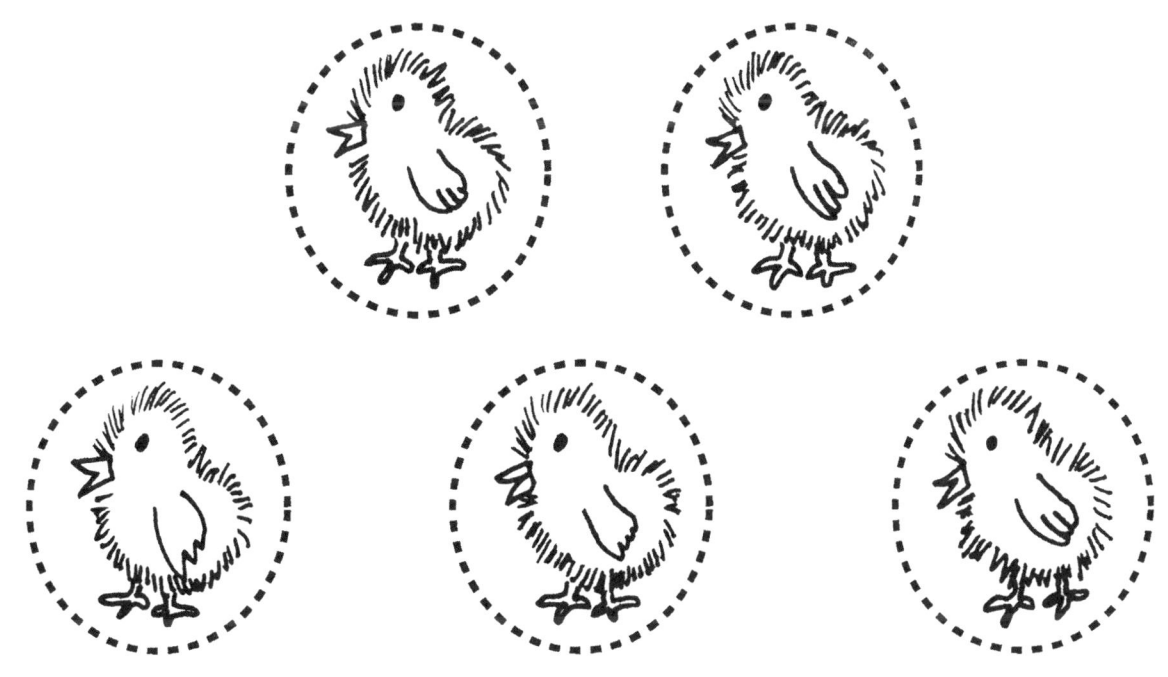

169

Good Eggs!

Good Eggs!

Make a bulletin board with the title "Good Eggs." Reproduce worksheet for each child. Have the child color and cut out eggs. As the child completes his homework, can say a new sound, or needs positive reinforcement, write something special on one of his eggs and allow him to place it on the bulletin board.

> Ex: John can say the "SH" sound.
> Brian did his homework.
> Latasha helped clean up.

Yes/No Sentence Completion

Reproduce worksheet for child. Use in conjunction with Yes/No questions or Sentence Completion (page 164). Have the child color an egg when his response is correct.

Fill the Basket

Obtain a real Easter basket. Reproduce worksheet for each child. Have child color and cut out eggs. As child responds to questions correctly, he can put an egg in the basket.

Other Suggestions/Activities

- Make an Easter Egg tree. Use a branch from a tree and place in a bucket of sand. Have child color and cut out eggs. Punch hole in top. Hang from tree branch with yarn.

Good Eggs!

Easter - Worksheet 72

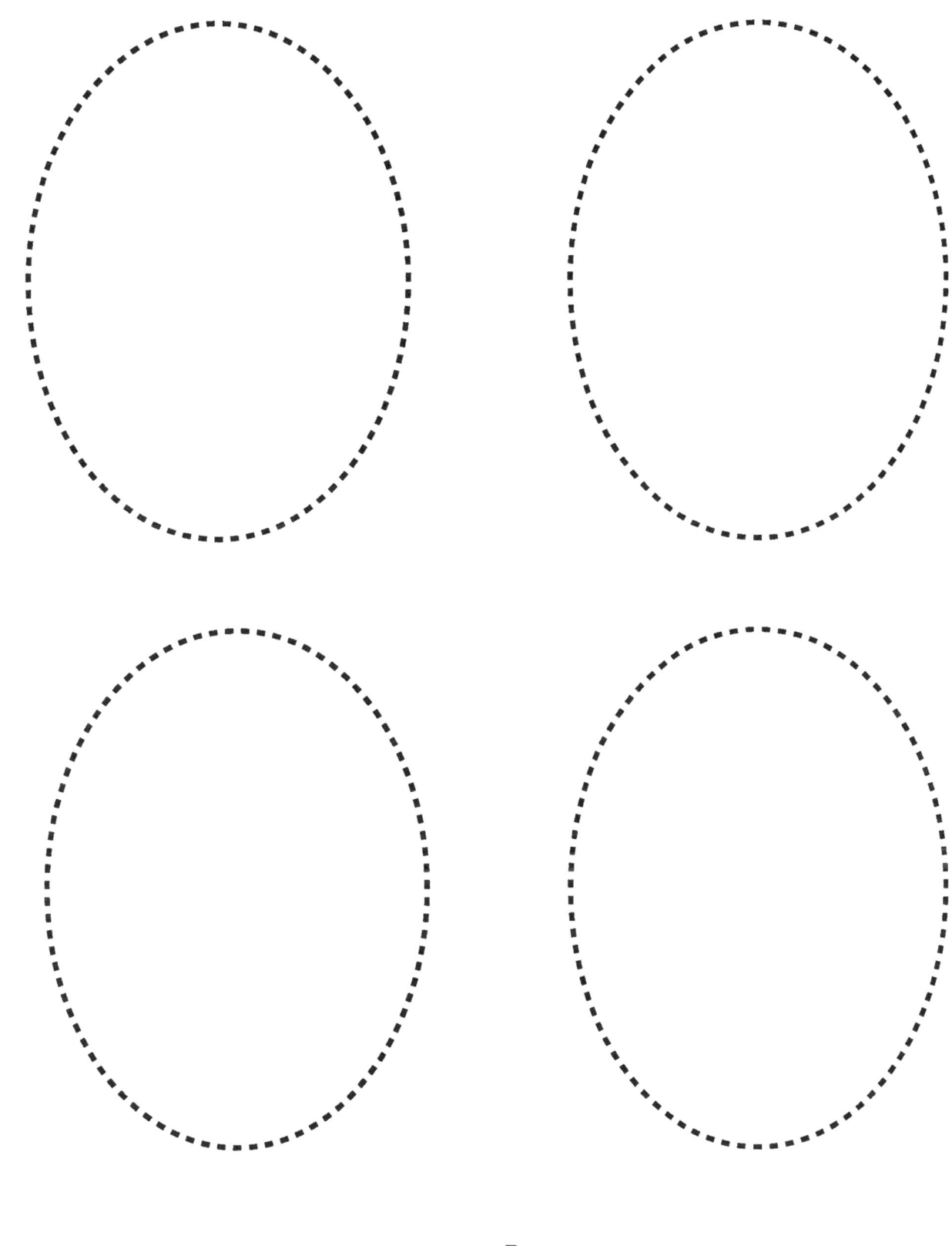

Name _____ Date _____

171

Flower Time

Easter - Worksheet 73

Instructor: Discuss how plants grow in the spring. Example:

"In the spring, many plants begin to grow. Trees grow green leaves. The grass turns green. Flowers begin to bloom. Spring brings warmer weather. Plants need sunshine to grow. Plants also need water to grow. It rains in the spring.

Sequence Activity

Have the child color and cut out each picture. Then, the child can put the pictures in order and paste on a piece of construction paper.

Listen and Say

Instructor: This activity allows the child to listen to a question and them immediately respond. Read the statement then ask the child the question.

1. In spring, many plants begin to grow.
   When do plants begin to grow?

2. Trees grow green leaves in spring.
   What do trees grow in spring?

3. Flowers begin to bloom in spring.
   What begins to bloom in spring?

4. Spring brings warm weather and rain.
   What is the weather like in spring?

5. Plants need sunshine and rain to grow.
   What do plants need to grow?

Other Suggestions/Activities

- Have the child plant a seed and observe growth on a daily basis.

- Have the child tell a short story about the three pictures.

172

Flower Time

Easter - Worksheet 73

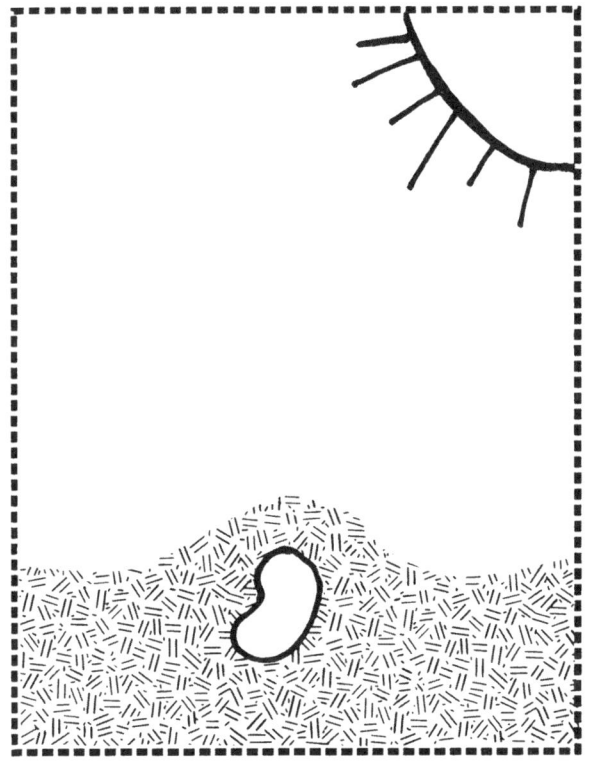

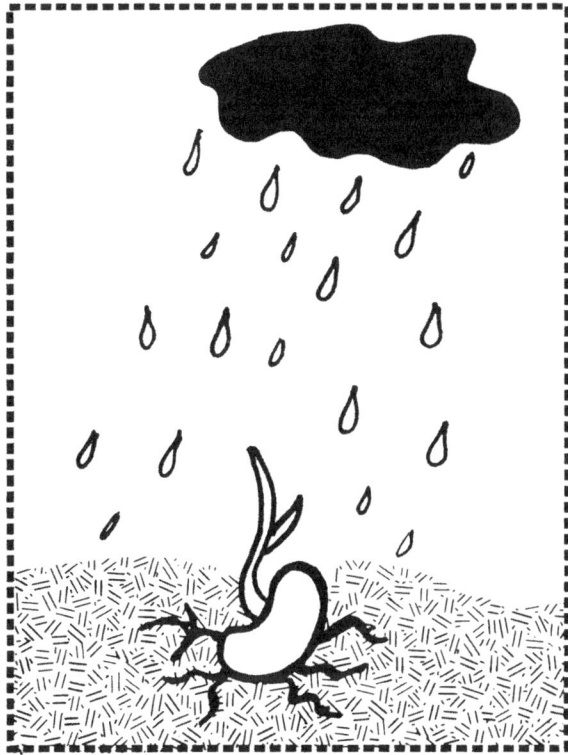

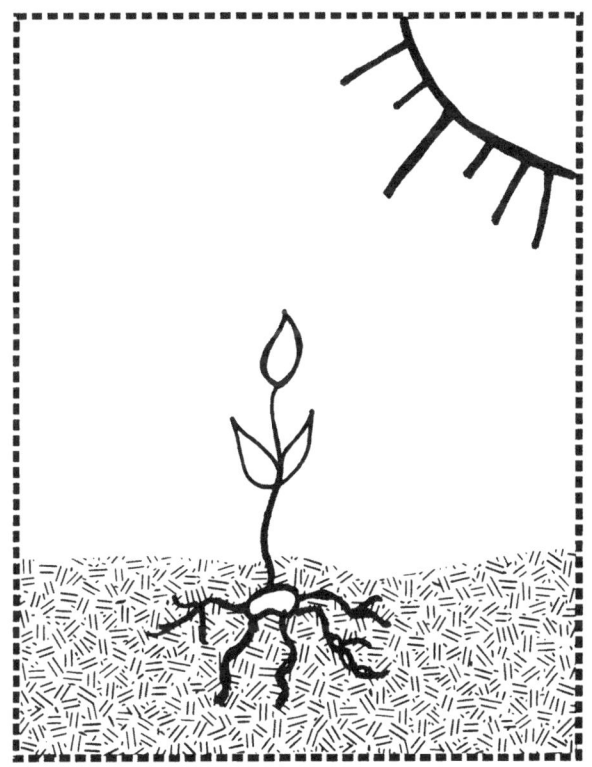

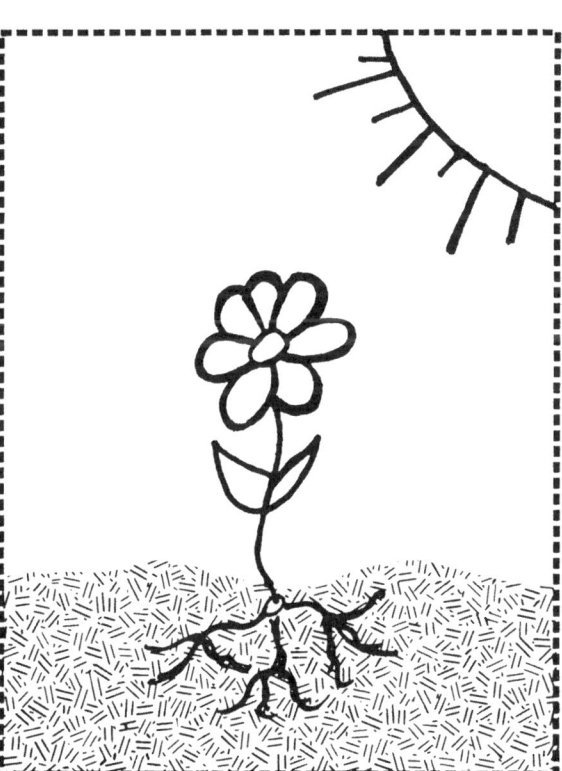

Easter Story

Instructor: Read "A Spring Surprise" to child. If possible, use props to assist in attending skills. (Have an Easter basket filled with eggs, a toy rabbit, turtle, or chick nearby.)

Storytime

Reproduce stick puppets (page 177). Have the child color, cut out, and paste on a tongue depressor or popsicle stick. Use while telling the story or have children hold up a stick puppet when they hear the name of their character in the story.

Use the stick puppets and have the child retell a part of the story.

Other Suggestions/Activities

- Read one paragraph at a time and ask "WH" questions.

   Ex: Paragraph 1
     What is the boy's name?
     What is the weather like?
     What is his friend's name?

- Have the child draw a picture about the story and tell about his picture.

A Spring Surprise

Characters: Keith, Renee, Uncle Bob, turtle

Keith gets up early one spring morning. The sun is shining. It has rained during the night. Keith gets dressed quickly and goes outside for a walk. Renee, Keith's friend, is outside too.

"Come look at this baby turtle," says Renee. "The shell has pretty colors," says Keith. "The hard shell protects the turtle from danger," says Renee.

Keith's Uncle Bob comes outside. He sees the turtle. "That is a box turtle," says Uncle Bob. "Box turtles are land turtles. The turtle is very quiet," says Renee. "I wonder what he would say if he could talk," says Uncle Bob. "Help! I'm stuck in this shell," says Keith. Everyone laughs at Keith's joke. "Maybe if we are very quiet," says Uncle Bob, "the turtle will come out of its shell."

Keith, Renee and Uncle Bob sit quietly and watch the turtle. Finally, the turtle sticks out its head and begins to walk very slowly. They watch for awhile until the turtle walks into the woods by Renee's house.

Uncle Bob says, "The weather outside is very nice. Spring is a time of the year when many things grow. The weather gets warmer. We get sunshine and rain. Flowers start to bloom, the leaves are growing on the trees, and the grass is turning green." "Baby turtles are born in the spring," says Renee.

"Easter is this weekend," says Keith. "I'm going to dye some Easter eggs. Can you stay and help?" he asks Renee. "Oh, yes," says Renee. "I love to dye Easter eggs!" Uncle Bob, Keith, and Renee walk back to the house.

Uncle Bob has boiled the eggs and they are cool enough to dye. Keith and Renee fill five cups with water. Next, they mix the egg dye and vinegar in the water. They have yellow, green, red, purple, and blue. They put an egg in each cup. After waiting a few minutes, they take the eggs out. "Easter eggs are so very pretty," says Renee. "My favorite is red," says Keith. "I like blue," says Renee. They let the eggs dry.

"We have an Easter egg hunt every year," says Keith. "It's fun to look for Easter eggs," says Renee. "You have to look in the flowers and grass, under bushes, and behind trees."

"I like the surprises, too," says Uncle Bob. "If you look out our kitchen window, you may see something surprising." Keith and Renee look out the window and on a branch in a small bush is a bird's nest. "Wow!" says Keith. "Look at those tiny eggs," says Renee. "They are blue!" Those are a robin's eggs," says Uncle Bob. "We will have to wait awhile to see the baby birds." "I'm going to look at them everyday," says Keith.

"Let's go look for our turtle again," says Keith. "Maybe we could take him for a walk," says Renee. "Let's go ask him," says Keith "and see what he says!"

Easter Story - Stick Puppets

Easter - Worksheet 74

Instructions: Have child color then cut out each character. Paste each character to the end of a tongue depressor or popsicle stick.

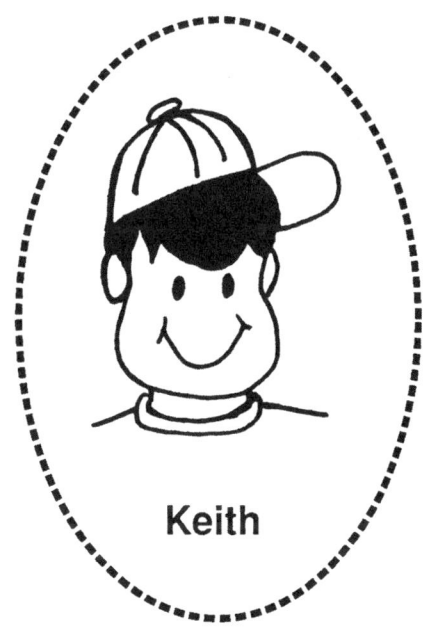

Keith

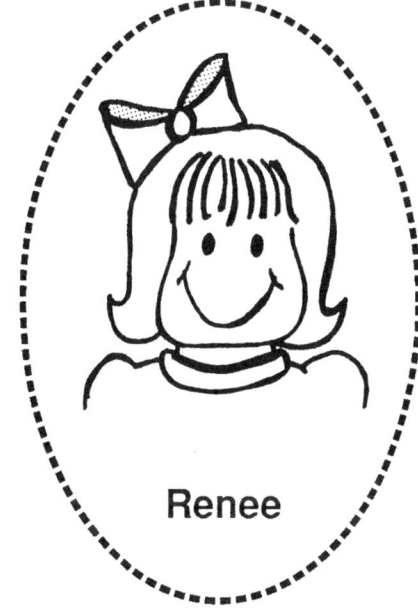

Renee

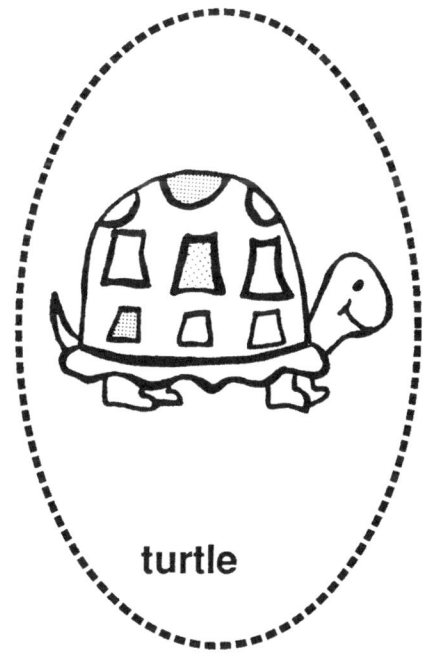

turtle

Uncle Bob

Rhyming Time

Instructor: Reproduce stick puppets (Page 179). Have child color and cut out. Paste each character to the end of a tongue depressor or popsicle stick.

The Turtle

There's the turtle,
In his shell.
What does he think?
It's hard to tell.

Easter Bunny

The Easter Bunny,
Hops, hops, hops,
And at my house,
He stops, stops, stops.

Easter Eggs

Let's dye some eggs,
For me and you.
I like red and yellow,
Green and purple, too.

Spring

In the spring,
The birds sing.
The flowers bloom,
The world's in tune.

Chick

The little chick,
Is a fluffy fellow.
He says cheep, cheep,
And is bright yellow.

Instructor: Have the child learn one poem and recite it using a stick puppet.

Other Suggestions/Activities

- Sentence Completion: Read a poem and leave off the last word in a line. Have the child complete the line by saying the word.

- Rewrite a poem on large chart paper. Have the child draw a picture to go with the poem. Place on bulletin board.

Rhyming Time - Stick Puppets

Easter - Worksheet 75

Instructions: Have child color then cut out each character. Paste each character to the end of a tongue depressor or popsicle stick.

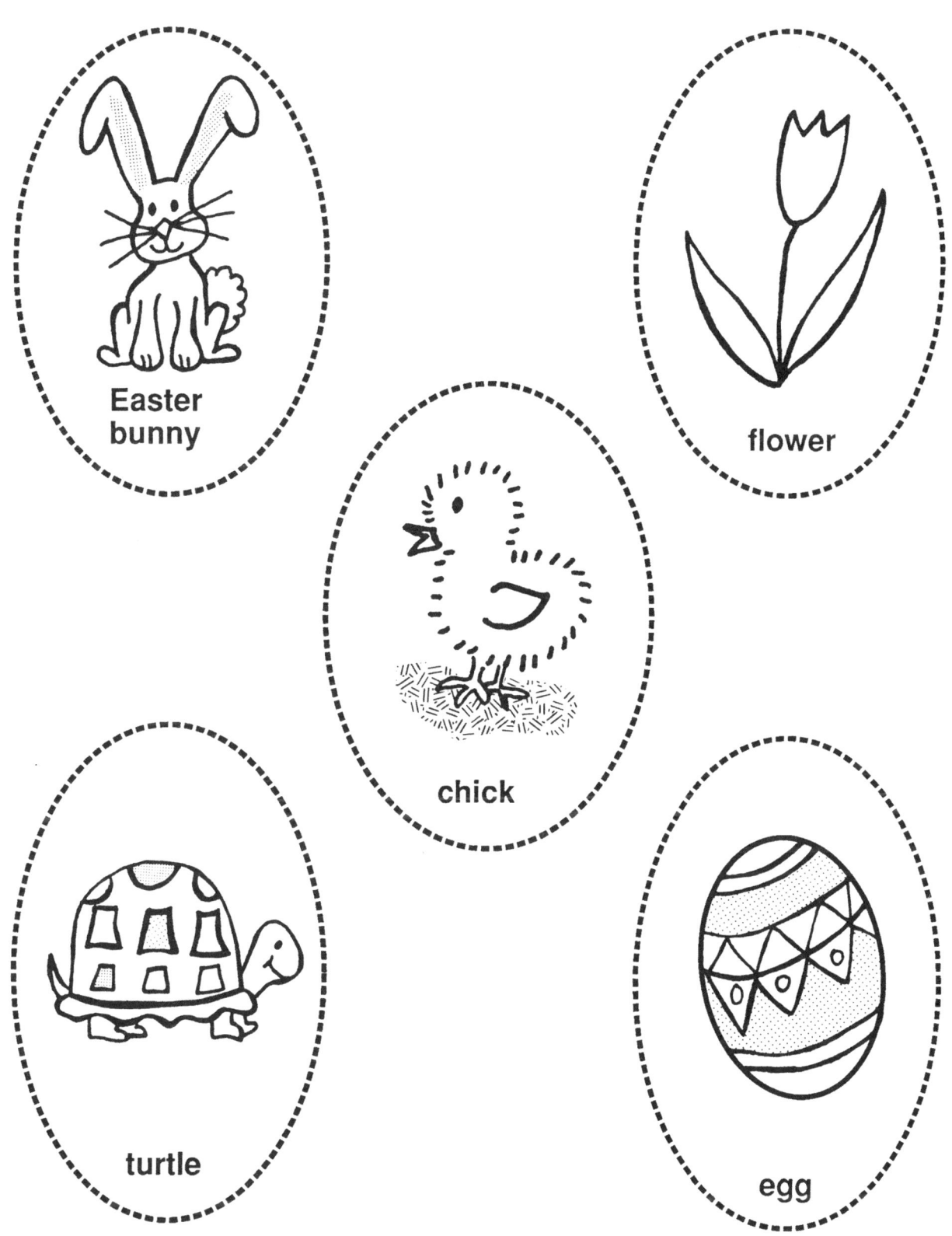

Easter
bunny

flower

chick

turtle

egg

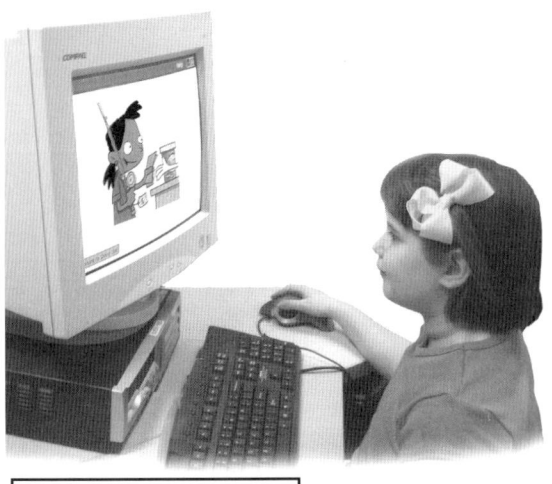

Auditory Memory for Quick Stories
Interactive CD-ROM/Fun Sheets Combo

Grades PreK-5

Created by Sharon G. Webber
Written by Keri Brown
Formatted by Mark Strait

Improve your child's listening skills step-by-step with these 30 delightful short stories and follow-up comprehension questions. Increase the difficulty level of the program as your students progress. Here's what you get:

Interactive CD-ROM

- Student uses program alone or with teacher.
- 30 illustrated narrated stories with six follow-up questions.
- Four levels of increasing difficulty for gradual improvement.
- Play scene by scene, one-half story, or entire story.
- Automatic feedback for correct/incorrect answers.
- Data-tracking for an unlimited number of students.
- Color and black and white fun sheets.
- Good Listening Awards.

Reproducible Workbook

- Ideal for home follow-up.
- Identical 30 stories, plus eight additional questions per story.
- Perforated pages for easy copying and pocket folders for storage.

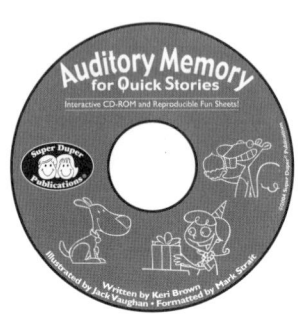

System Requirements

Windows®
- Intel Pentium II or equivalent
- Microsoft Windows® 98, ME, 2000, or XP
- 64 MB RAM
- 10 MB free disk space
- CD-ROM drive
- Sound card and color monitor

Macintosh®
- Power Macintosh G3
- Mac OS 9 or OSX
- 128 MB RAM
- 10 MB hard drive space
- CD-ROM drive
- Sound card and color monitor

#AMLQ-110
Auditory Memory for Quick Stories

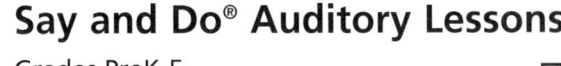

Auditory Memory for Rhyming Words in Sentences
Fun Deck®

Grades K-3

by Sharon G. Webber

Listen carefully. "The duck is driving a truck." Now you say it. Improve your students' listening and phonemic awareness skills with these 54 delightful cards (38 short vowel and 16 long vowel sounds).

#FD-69
Auditory Memory in Sentences Fun Deck®

Say and Do® Auditory Lessons

Grades PreK-5

by Diane Hyde

Improve your students' auditory processing at two skill levels, beginner and advanced, with this 60-page reproducible. Lesson sheets target twenty areas of listening development.

- **Auditory Association** - WH questions, Auditory Closure, Parts to Whole, If-Then, What's Wrong with the Sentence, Listening for Main Idea, Similarities & Differences.
- **Auditory Discrimination** - Rhyming, Syllable Awareness, Identification/Discrimination of Initial Sounds in Words, Identification & Discrimination of Final Sounds in Words, Sound Blending.
- **Auditory Memory** - Memory for Words, Memory for Short Sentences, Memory for Long Sentences, Memory for Poems, Listening for Details.
- **Auditory Reception** - Yes/No Questions, Which Is, True/False.

#BK-313
"Say and Do"® Auditory Lessons

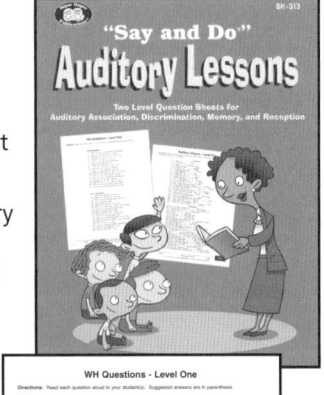

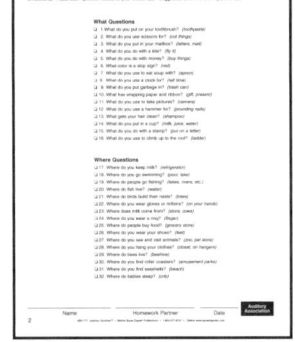

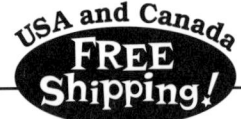

Artic Quickies®

Reproducible Photo Fun Sheets with Color CD-ROM Fun Sheets for S, R, L, K, G, F, SH, CH, TH & S/R/L Blends!

All Ages

If someone told you that you could get reproducible articulation photo fun sheets with color CD-ROM fun sheets, all for under $10, would you believe it? Well, it's true, compliments of Super Duper®'s brand new *Artic Quickies®* series.

Artic Quickies® is really two photo-based products in one - a reproducible workbook and a CD-ROM - full of handy, multi-purpose funsheets. *Quickies®* takes the 28 photo-words found in the *Artic Photos Fun Decks®* and adds in another 28 bonus photo-words to create lively activity pages. Directions on these pages allow you to choose the appropriate level of articulation practice - word, phrase, or sentence.

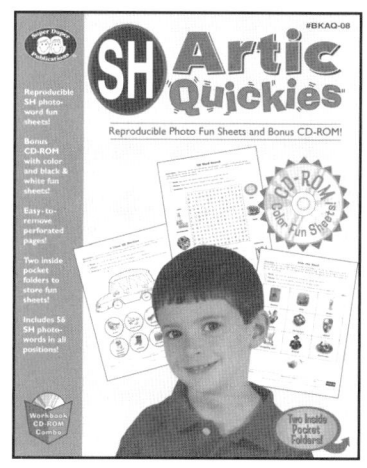

Reproducible Fun Sheets plus Color CD-ROM Fun Sheets!

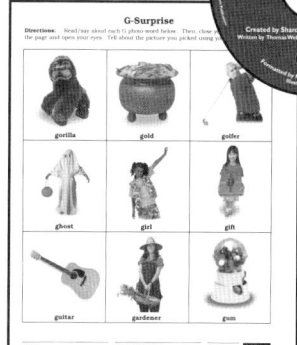

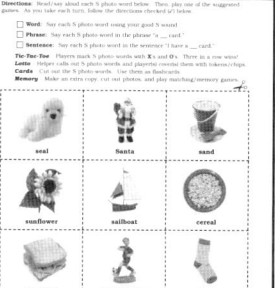

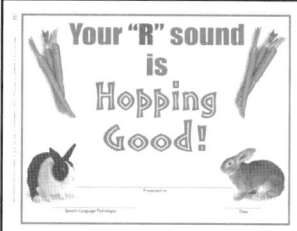

CD Includes Bonus Awards!

S Artic Quickies®.....#BKAQ-01
R Artic Quickies®.....#BKAQ-02
L Artic Quickies®.....#BKAQ-03
S Blends Quickies®..#BKAQ-04
R Blends Quickies®..#BKAQ-05
L Blends Quickies®..#BKAQ-06
SH Artic Quickies®.....#BKAQ-08
CH Artic Quickies®.....#BKAQ-09
TH Artic Quickies®.... #BKAQ-10
K Artic Quickies®.....#BKAQ-11
G Artic Quickies®.....#BKAQ-12
F Artic Quickies®.....#BKAQ-13

Early Articulation Roundup™!

Fun Sheets for B, D, F, G, H, K, M, N, NG, P, T, V, W, and Y!

Grades PreK - 2

by Beverly Foster and Stacy Lynn Foster

You will need your spurs and a ten-gallon hat for this *Rinky Link* book with over 1300 fun-filled illustrations for 14 early developing sounds: B, D, F, G, H, K, M, N, NG, P, T, V, W & Y. Each sound is in the initial, medial, and final positions (except ng, w, and y). You get 214 pages of humorous illustrations where children can "round up" their very own pictures and keep them on the *Rinky Link* plastic ring (24 included!). Activities for each sound are...

- *Oral Motor Exercises/Articulation Practice:* Teach the target sound (kuh...kuh...sound).

- *Auditory Discrimination Pairs:* A listening activity that helps the child identify the error sound (key-tea).

- *Syllable Practice:* Practice target sounds in syllables with short/long vowels (ka in "cat" and ka in "cake").

- *Word, Phrase, and Sentence Pictures:* Practice each target sound at the word, phrase, and sentence level.

- *Helper's Log:* A helpful Homework Helper's chart.

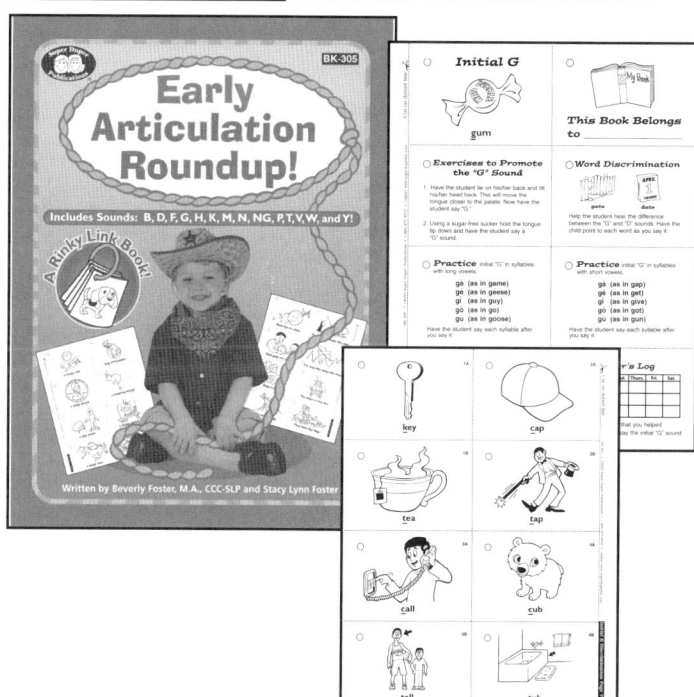

You also receive target book covers, awards, a progress chart, and a parent letter. So, rustle up some early sounds today!

#BK-305
Early Articulation Roundup™!

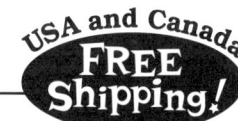

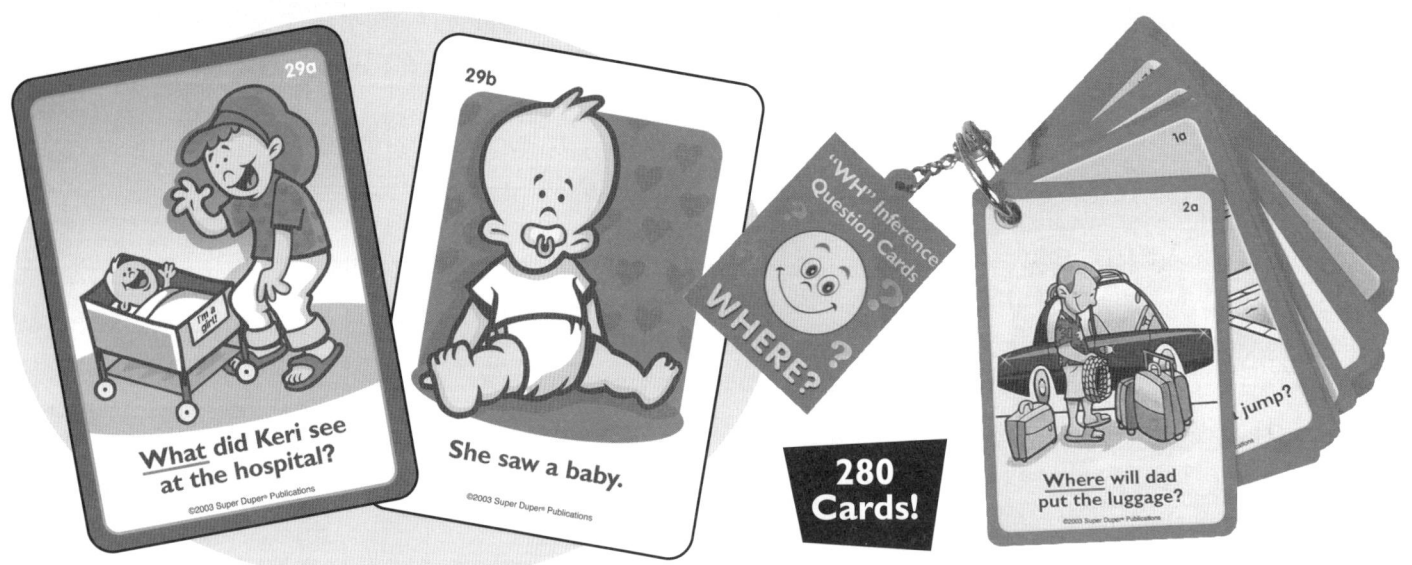

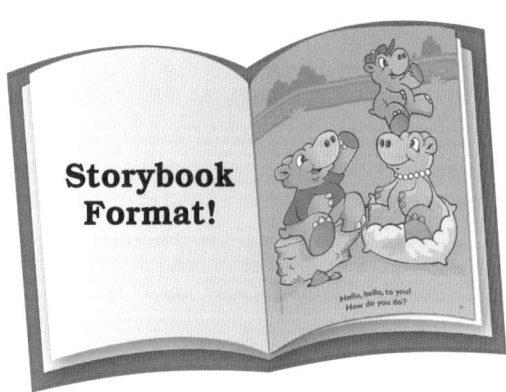
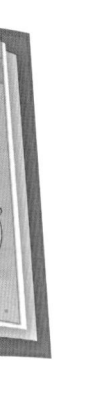
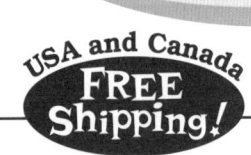
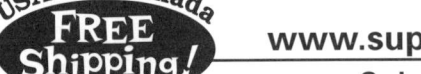

Notes

_____

_____

_____

_____

_____

_____

_____

_____

_____

_____

_____

_____

_____

_____

_____

Notes